THE
FOODS of Love

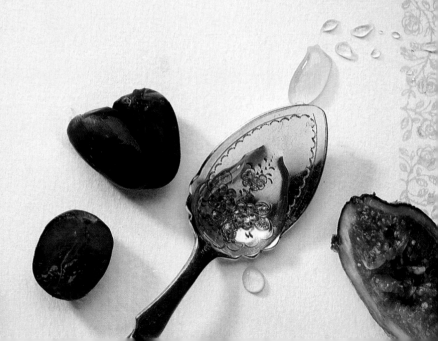

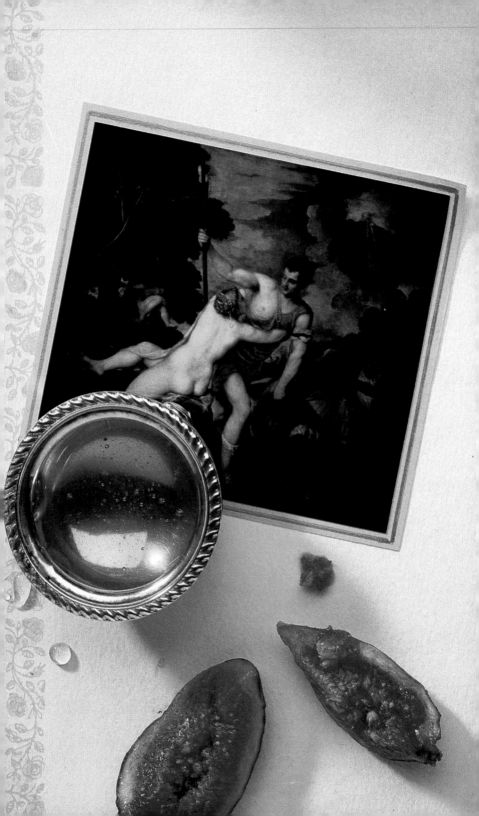

THE
FOODS of Love

Containing the DELIGHTS, *Vertues,*
Magickal *Properties &* SECRET
Recipes for all manner of
exquisite LOVE POTIONS *&*
proven **Aphrodisiacs**

MAX de ROCHE

DORLING KINDERSLEY · LONDON

A DORLING KINDERSLEY BOOK

EDITOR Susan Berry
DESIGNED BY Sara Nunan/Bridgewater Design Ltd
PHOTOGRAPHY Guy Ryecart
ARTWORK Jenny Millington

MANAGING EDITOR Daphne Razazan
ART DIRECTOR Anne-Marie Bulat

First published in Great Britain in 1990
by Dorling Kindersley Limited
9 Henrietta Street, London WC2E 8PS

NOTE: While every effort has been made by the author and publishers
to ensure that the commonly available ingredients discussed in this book
are safe (unless otherwise stated), anyone wishing to take the more
unusual aphrodisiacs would be advised to consult an appropriate medical
or herbal authority beforehand. Neither the author nor the publishers
can take any responsibility for the misuse of any of the ingredients, or for
their efficacy or possible adverse side effects.

British Library Cataloguing in Publication Data
De Roche, Max
    Foods of love.
    1. Food: Aphrodisiacs: Recipes
    I. Title
    641.5

ISBN 0-86318-495-2

Typeset by CST (Hove) Ltd
Printed and bound by
Graphicom in Italy

CONTENTS

Introduction 6

LOVE POTIONS
—— 10 ——

THE FOODS OF LOVE
—— 26 ——

MENUS FOR ROMANTIC ENCOUNTERS
—— 74 ——

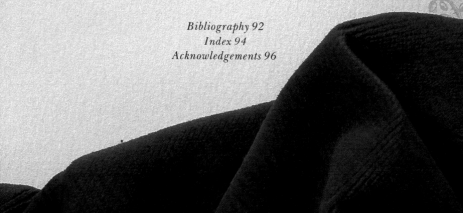

INTRODUCTION

YIN

*"The causes of enjoyment are six in
number: the fire of ardent love,
superabundance of sperm, proximity of the
loved one, beauty of face, exciting viands,
and contact."*

THE PERFUMED GARDEN

THIS MAY SOUND rather carnal, but in fact the carnal and
the spiritual are inseparable. Two lines of John Donne's
in the *Extasie* express it succinctly and accurately:
*"Love's mysteries in soules doe grow
but yet the body is his booke."*
Man has been concerned with love, and with aphrodisiacs,
for as long as our history has been recorded. In all cultures,
people have been concocting love potions and philtres to
ensnare and entrance the opposite sex, and to improve their
performance in the act itself. The name "love potion" suggests a magic substance that, having been swallowed, sends
lovers off into new realms of delight. Many classical aphrodisiacs are long gone, ridiculed and discredited. Rhinoceros
horn, for example, has absolutely nothing to justify it, and
the universal myth of mandrake (in any event highly poisonous) has declined into obscurity. Alcohol, useful to shift
minor inhibitions, was put in its place accurately by Shake-
speare in *Macbeth*: *"It provoketh desire, but takes away the
performance"*.

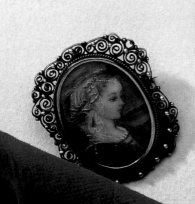

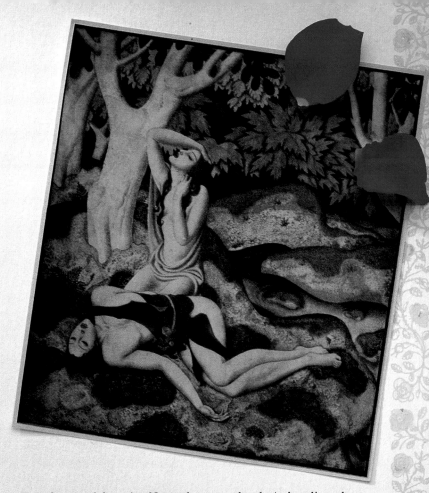

For the word love itself, we have to thank Aphrodite, the Greek Goddess of Love, who sprang naked from the foaming sea near Cythera in the sixth century BC, and ever since has been worshipped as a fertility goddess. Aphrodite represents a sexuality free from ambivalence, anxiety and self-consciousness. Her cult came to Greece from the East, but Praxiteles, the fourth-century BC sculptor, gave her such an evocative form that she became, for Western civilization, the embodiment of primordial femininity.

It seems difficult to believe, to those educated in an orthodox Christian background, that "love" itself was a religion in Greece at that time, but, as Kenneth Clark explains in *Civilization*, "*perhaps no religion ever again incorporated physical passion so naturally that all who saw Aphrodite felt that the instincts they shared with the beasts, they also shared with the gods*".

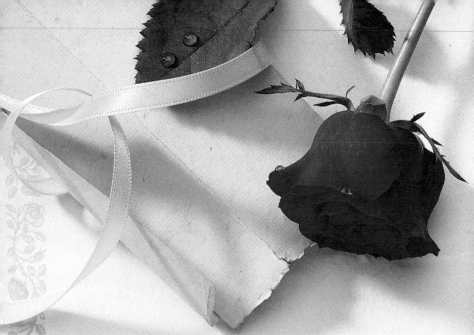

This Greek religion of the fifth century BC was not unique. The Hindus have always considered love to be sacramental, the human counterpart of Creation. To them, sex is the coupling of *Parusha* (master) with *Prariti* (energy) and is deified by the union of Shiva and Shakti, which they believe created the world. The symbol of Shiva is the *lingam* (phallus) and the symbol of Shakti is the *yoni* (vagina). This is all contained in the *Rig Veda* or *Hymn of Creation*:

> *"Desire then arose,*
> *Desire which was the earliest seed of Spirit,*
> *the Bond of Being".*

The philosophy of the Tao in China, with its governing principles of Yin (female), Yang (male) and Chi (spirit and energy), similarly relates sexual union to the cosmos, maintaining that a balance between Yin and Yang can cause, when perfect, a vibration similar to the rhythms of the universe.

Although the reasons for attraction and desire are almost as much a mystery today as they were in ancient times, we do know that the spur for sexual desire begins in the brain – in the hypothalamus, which also governs our appetites for food and drink. It does seem that all these activities are closely related and can influence both the awakening and the fulfilment of desire. But good and happy sexual relations are far more than simple sexual athleticism.

The current mythology of ceaseless male sexuality is sadly fictitious. Men sometimes worry that the exquisite magic erection may not materialize and Zulu warriors in the 19th century carried amulets to ensure that they would have a good erection after battle. As Aristotle pointed out, if there is no strength in you, aphrodisiacs will be useless. Undoubtedly, fitness and virility, good health and fertility, go hand in hand.

The *Kama Sutra* gives invaluable advice on achieving a happy sex life:

> *"Do not have a stomach full of food and drink, or*
> *you will have apoplexy and gout . . . A man should*
> *eat strengthening foods, such as aromatic plants,*
> *meat, honey and eggs. A robust constitution is*
> *indispensable for copulation, but, above all, play*
> *with her lovingly, until she is excited and full*
> *of desire."*

The "foods of love" are many and varied, and in this book I have listed those with the greatest aphrodisiac properties, together with recipes for using them to best advantage. The first chapter describes some love potions, philtres and powders that can often be added to these foods to give them extra sparkle, the second details the ingredients with magical properties, and the last gives a selection of menus designed to enhance various romantic encounters.

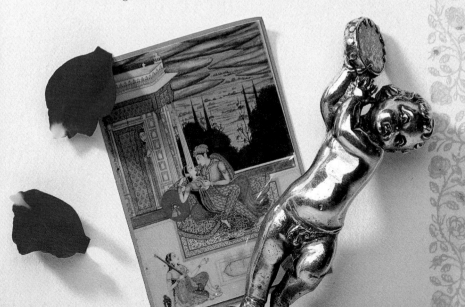

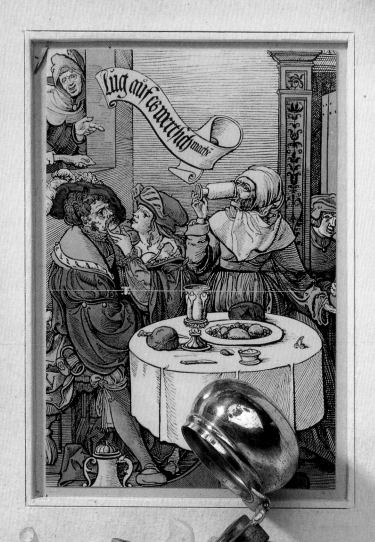

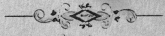

LOVE POTIONS

THESE LOVE POTIONS are for lovers, to keep them ecstatic when all is well or to bring some pleasures if times are stressful, when good love-making may be in the balance.

The recipes and suggestions in this chapter have been taken from Indian, Chinese and Arabic texts, and medieval manuscripts, among other sources. To make them at home, you will need a pestle and mortar and some storage jars, as well as the usual kitchen equipment. A food processor or liquidizer and an electric coffee grinder will make the work easier.

Many of these love potions may be used as additions to other recipes. Experiment with small quantities – the tastes are generally agreeable or indiscernible. Recipes marked with * are suitable for home use; the others are included for their curiosity value.

GINSENG SYRUP*

Ginseng is one of the most potent aphrodisiacs and is discussed in detail on pages 52–3. It is available, ready prepared and in various forms, from health food shops. This syrup is made using the root, and can be added to any vegetable dishes.

2 LARGE GINSENG ROOTS, OR 4 SMALL ONES, CUT UP FINE

300 ml (½ pt) WATER

45 ml (3 tbsp) SAKE OR VODKA

Pound the ginseng roots in a mortar and then place them in an earthenware casserole with the liquid. Heat in a low oven (140°C/275°F/gas mark 1) for two hours, then leave overnight in the oven at the lowest possible temperature. The next morning, strain and bottle the liquid.

Store in a cool place. It will keep for up to a month.

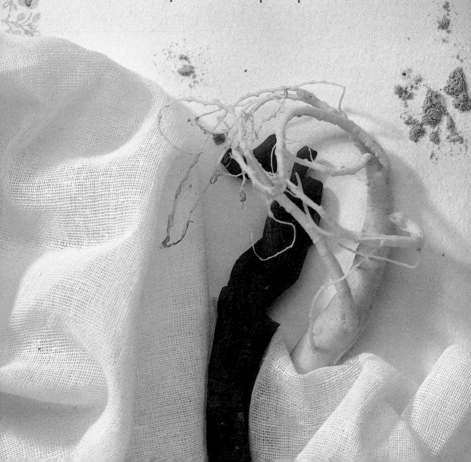

SATYRION

*An "Electuary of Satyrion" was made
from the nectar of wild orchid (Orchis
mascula) squeezed into goat's milk
"which hath a great force to provide the
desire for coition and doth egregiously
excite both sexes therewith",
according to John Partridge,
physician to Charles I.*

To make this aphrodisiac,
which had also been highly regarded
by the Greeks and Romans, you first have to
find 20 stalks of *Orchis mascula* (which can be found growing wild in Europe). Press the flowers and squeeze out the
nectar into 600 ml (1 pt) of warm Greek yogurt or goat's milk.

This is a general-purpose potion and can be added in
small quantities to virtually any dish or eaten for breakfast,
to start the day properly.

MARROW BONE JELLY*

*This very nourishing jelly is a marvellous restorative and pick-me-up.
It is best served in a meat dish like Oyster Beef Slices (see page 43),
where it will add to the general aphrodisiac properties.*

Collect several 12.5 cm (5 in) beef and veal marrow bones
from your butcher. Stand them upright and cut them in half
with a cleaver or sharp chopper. Take out the marrow and
simmer it with a little dry white wine. Stir in just sufficient
aspic powder to make it into a jelly.

Store the jelly in a labelled glass jar in the refrigerator. It
will keep for 3-4 days.

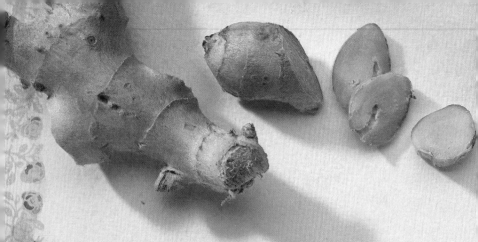

PEKING LIQUOR AND ELIXIR*

This is a recipe that every Chinese chef knows, as did his grandfather, and his grandfather before him. The Chinese have been concerned with aphrodisiacs for thousands of years, or certainly with cooking that gives deep satisfaction long after the taste is forgotten, as it stimulates the vital areas of the body.

1.5 litres (3 pt) WATER

900 g (2 lb) KNUCKLE OF PORK, WHOLE

450 g (1 lb) PORK BELLY, CUT INTO 4 PIECES

½ CHICKEN, BONED AND CHOPPED

300 ml (½ pt) CHINESE YELLOW WINE (OR DRY SHERRY)

100 ml (7 tbsp) SOY SAUCE

30 ml (2 tbsp) SUGAR

3 THIN SLICES ROOT GINGER

Put the water into a large casserole and add the meat. Boil for 5 minutes. Pour off all the water. Add half the wine, the soy sauce, sugar and ginger and mix together.

Place the covered casserole in the oven and cook at 140°C/ 275°F/gas mark 1 for 3½ hours.

Add another 125 ml (¼ pint) water and the rest of the wine, and stir. Remove all the solids and use for other meals. Collect the liquid in a bowl and remove the fat. Strain and cool.

The resultant liquor should be stored in a jar marked "Peking Liquor". The jelly is "Peking Elixir". Both will keep for up to 4 days in the refrigerator.

NUT AND POMEGRANATE GOLD*

Spread on Bath Olivers or on rye biscuits, this mixture is invigorating, sustaining and inspiring.

2 POMEGRANATES

30 ml (2 tbsp) GROUND ALMONDS

15 ml (1 tbsp) SESAME SEEDS

15 ml (1 tbsp) PUMPKIN SEEDS

15 ml (1 tbsp) PINE KERNELS

30 ml (2 tbsp) SAKE

Remove the skins of the pomegranates and cut the fruit into horizontal slices so that the flesh can be removed, leaving the pith. Shred the pith finely, and add to it the ground almonds, sesame and pumpkin seeds, and the pine kernels. Grind the mixture with the sake and 30 ml (2 tbsp) of pomegranate fruit flesh.

The mixture will keep for up to a week in a refrigerator.

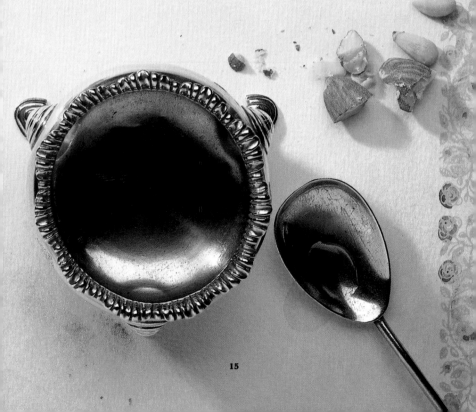

Cardamom Syrup*

This recipe was advocated by John Partridge, King Charles I's physician. Both Partridge and the King spent some time at the court of Louis XIV at a time when love potions and invigorating syrups were all the rage.

15 ml (1 tbsp) EACH OF CARDAMOM, CINNAMON AND NETTLE SEED

SLICE OF ROOT GINGER, FINELY CHOPPED

15 ml (1 tbsp) OF CHOPPED SEA SPURGE
(*Euphorbia paralias*) – IF AVAILABLE

125 ml (4 fl oz) WATER

125 ml (4 fl oz) HONEY

Mix the dry ingredients with a little of the water to make a paste, add the rest of the water and liquidize. Simmer for 1 hour and then add the honey.

Store the syrup in a labelled jar or eat immediately with apricots or peaches.

Apricot Gold*

This has been known for hundreds of years in China, and there are several versions of it. Lao Tsze, the legendary Chinese philosopher, believed in it, and today dieticians agree that it is remarkably full of vitamins, as well as a great restorative of fertility. It is also a provocative and delicious love potion. It is very easy to prepare and can even be made with tinned apricots if fresh ones are not available.

Emulsify the apricots (stone them first if using fresh) in a liquidizer and add royal jelly in the proportions of 50 of fruit to 5 of royal jelly.

It is good for breakfast, or as a dessert for lunch or dinner.

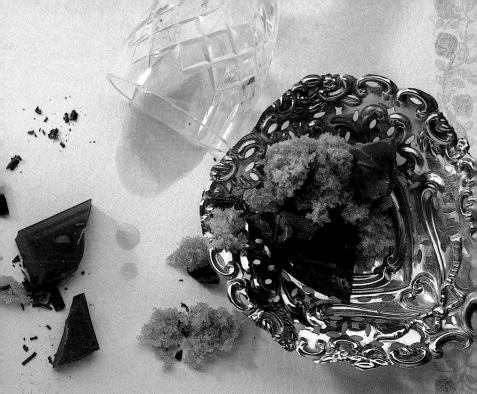

Chocolate Benedictine*

The chocolate, sugar and the liqueur combine to give an instant source of energy.

100 g (4 oz) BROWN SUGAR

150 ml (¼ pt) WATER

100 g (4 oz) BITTER CHOCOLATE

4 EGG YOLKS

2.5 ml (½ tsp) ALLSPICE

15 ml (1 tbsp) BLACK COFFEE

30 ml (2 tbsp) BENEDICTINE

300 ml (½ pt) WHIPPED CREAM

Melt the sugar in the water over a low heat. Melt the chocolate in a bowl over a pan of boiling water, whisk the eggs into the chocolate and stir in the allspice and the sugar syrup. Allow to cool, then add the black coffee and Benedictine, and fold in the cream. Pour into individual small dishes and chill.

It can also be frozen and eaten as ice-cream, if preferred.

BANANA SYRUP*

*Jamaican limbo dancers are reputed to get some of their zest from this.
Add it to fruit salad.*

8 BANANAS

DASH OF JAMAICAN ALLSPICE

50 g (2 OZ) BROWN SUGAR

Bake the bananas in their skins in a moderate oven until tender. (Alternatively, stew the bananas for about 20 minutes.) Remove the fruit flesh and use it for a sweet. Scrape the insides of the skins and mix the scrapings with the allspice and sugar. Dissolve the sugar over low heat with 15 ml (1 tbsp) water, to make a syrup.

WALNUT CREAM*

*Although this sounds bland and innocuous,
walnuts were regarded as a symbol of
fecundity in both Greek and Roman times,
and were thrown at weddings to the
children by the bridegroom, who
presumably felt he was no longer in need
of such symbols.*

225 g (½ lb) BROKEN WALNUTS

300 ml (½ pt) GOAT'S MILK

45 ml (3 tbsp) HONEY

YOLKS OF 4 RAW EGGS

Chop the walnuts into small pieces and simmer them in the goat's milk until they soften and the liquid is thick. Liquidize the mixture with the honey and the egg yolks. The consistency should be very thick.

Walnut cream makes a valuable addition to a quiet snack of prosciutto or pastrami.

It can be stored in the refrigerator for up to 2 days.

AMRUS *

This love potion comes from the South Pacific,
where it is still in use today.

6 RIPE MANGOES

200 ml (⅓ pt) MILK

15 ml (1 tbsp) SUGAR

BLACK PEPPER, TO SEASON

Cut the mangoes into quarters and scrape the flesh from the skin and the stone. Put the fruit in the blender, add the milk and sugar, and liquidize. Sprinkle with a little black pepper to taste. It will keep for up to 48 hours in the refrigerator.

CHAUCER'S LOVE DISH*

This comes from the "Legend of the Good Woman" and is included in
To the King's Taste, *the cookbook prepared for Richard II by Lorna Sass in the 14th century.*

60 ml (4 tbsp) DRIED CRUSHED ROSE PETALS

375 ml (12 fl oz) ALMOND MILK
(BLANCHED ALMONDS SOAKED IN MILK AND HONEY)

2.5 ml (½ tsp) CINNAMON

2.5 ml (½ tsp) GINGER

10 ml (2 tsp) RICE FLOUR

100 g (4 oz) FRESH DATES, MINCED

45 ml (3 tbsp) PINE KERNELS

TO GARNISH: FRESH ROSE PETALS

Soak the dried petals in almond milk for 10 minutes and then add the cinnamon and ginger. Cook for 5 minutes over a low heat. Blend the rice flour with a couple of tablespoonsful of cold water. Add it with the dates and pine kernels, stir well, and pour into two bowls. Decorate with the rose petals.

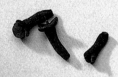

Arabian Delight

This comes from the Arabian Nights, *translated by Richard Burton, and is taken from the story of Ala-Al-Din Abu-Al. You could make it without the opium (illegal in most countries) and the mountain skink, for the value of the herbs and spices alone.*

"Two ounces of concentrated Roumi opium and equal parts of Chinese cubebs, cinnamon, cloves, cardamoms, ginger, white pepper, and mountain skink ... pounded together, boiled in olive oil, with three ounces of male frankincense, and a cup of coriander seed, macerating the whole and made into an electuary with Roumi bee honey.

Take with a spoon after supping, wash it down with a sherbet of rose conserve, but first sup off mutton and house pigeon seasoned and spiced."

Eryngo Jelly*

The following recipe is best added to eel or crab dishes, to achieve the greatest effect. Eryngo, or sea holly as it is sometimes known, grows wild by the coast in Europe and southern England, and can be grown in the garden.

1 ERYNGO PLANT *(Eryngium maritimum)*

YOLKS OF 4 RAW EGGS

45 ml (3 tbsp) MADEIRA

ASPIC POWDER

Wash the fleshy roots of the plant and cut them in 1 cm (½ in) pieces and simmer in a little water. Add the egg yolks and the Madeira and mix well. Stir in sufficient aspic powder, dissolved in boiling water, to turn it into a jelly.

It can be stored in the refrigerator for up to 2 days.

ABOVE ERYNGIUM MARITIMUM

CHICK PEA NECTAR*

This particular love potion could produce incredible results, according to the Ananga Ranga, *the ancient Indian "Art of Love".*

"Soak urid seeds (*Phaseolus mungo*) or chick peas in milk and sugar. Expose for three days to the rays of the sun. (Failing the sun, leave them overnight in a slow oven.) Reduce this to a powder, knead it into the form of cakes, and fry them in ghee. These should be eaten every morning and you will be able to enjoy a hundred women."

To make chick pea nectar at home, add four parts of macerated chick peas, one part of honey and one part of pounded onion to four parts of water. Simmer gently for about an hour, then sieve and liquidize the mixture.

It is prepared like this in Indian restaurants and usually added to vegetables.

CANTON LIQUOR*

The strained liquid that results from this recipe is clear Canton liquor, known to all Chinese chefs. Although the name changes from region to region, the liquor does not and it can be added to many recipes, such as stews and soups.

2.4 litres (4 pts) WATER

450 g (1 lb) SHIN BEEF, IN PIECES

900 g (2 lb) SPARE RIBS

700 g (1½ lb) HAM BONE

3 BEEF MARROW BONES

100 g (¼ lb) MINCED BEEF

100 g (¼ lb) MINCED CHICKEN BREAST

Place all the ingredients, apart from the minced beef and minced chicken, in a casserole. Simmer for 4 hours and skim off the fat. Add the minced beef and chicken. Simmer for 5 minutes and strain through a sieve. (You can use the meat for another dish.)

Bottle the liquid; store it in the refrigerator for up to 4 days.

Aqua Mirabilis*

*The 17th-century panacea for restoring vigour and refreshing the
spirit, Aqua Mirabilis comprised equal quantities of cinnamon,
ginger, thyme, rosemary, grated nutmeg and galingale root, all finely
ground and steeped in claret for a week. The wine was then strained,
and a glass taken daily.*

Diod Anfarwoleb*

*This is a Druid tonic to give you vigour and joy. Translated, the name
means "Draught of Immortality". It contains two of the seven herbs
sacred to the Druid religion, red clover and vervain, the latter being a
noted aphrodisiac.*

Prepare an infusion of chervil, heather, honeysuckle, red
clover and vervain by steeping a sprig of each in 300 ml (½
pt) water for a day. Strain it and take a tablespoonful night
and morning.

It will keep for up to a week in the refrigerator.

Quail's Egg Nectar*

*Raw egg yolks are full of protein, minerals and fats that get straight
into the bloodstream and act immediately on flagging libido. Eggs
feature heavily in Arabian love potions and in many French ones. This
recipe includes honey – in itself a powerful aphrodisiac – and is one of
the most palatable. As it is very protein-rich, it makes a wonderful
breakfast dish.*

10 QUAIL'S EGGS

125 ml (4 fl oz) HONEY

5 ml (1 tsp) SESAME OIL

10 ml (2 tsp) SAKE

This could not be simpler to make. Liquidize all the
ingredients except the sake until frothy. Add the sake and
pour into chilled glasses. Drink immediately.

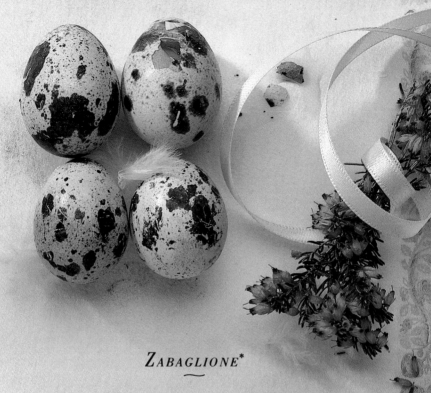

Zabaglione[*]

~

Italians have been giving themselves extra zest by drinking this delicious concoction since Renaissance times, and the French "sabayon" is similar in almost every respect. Even if the meal that precedes it is uninspiring, zabaglione will still work wonders. Although it has never been labelled an aphrodisiac, an aphrodisiac is what it is. Nutritive and exhilarating, and quick to prepare, it has an almost instant effect, with or without the addition of satyrion (see page 13).

YOLKS OF 3 RAW EGGS

45 ml (3 tbsp) HONEY

45 ml (3 tbsp) MADEIRA

15 ml (1 tbsp) COGNAC OR ARMAGNAC AND/OR SATYRION

Put all the ingredients in a bowl over a pan of hot water and beat with an electric mixer until light and fluffy. Serve hot. (If you wish, you can simply mix the ingredients cold but, of course, the mixture has a very different consistency, although the effect is similar.)

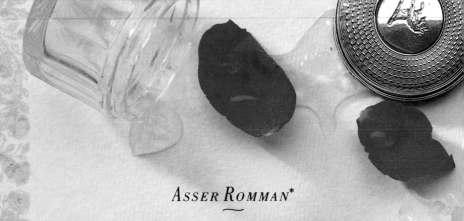

Asser Romman*

This Egyptian aphrodisiac is popular still.

2 LARGE POMEGRANATES

5 ml (1 tsp) ROSEWATER

300 ml (½ pt) ICED WATER

JUICE OF ½ LEMON

HONEY, TO TASTE

Remove the skin and seeds from the pomegranates and blend the fruit with the other ingredients in the liquidizer. It will keep for a few days in the refrigerator.

Chestnut and Ginger Delight*

A surprisingly potent combination, but too rich to be taken in large quantities.

4 EGG YOLKS

45 ml (3 tbsp) CASTER SUGAR

225 g (8 OZ) CHESTNUT PURÉE

50 g (2 OZ) FRESH GINGER, FINELY SLICED AND GROUND

60 ml (4 tbsp) COINTREAU

15 ml (1 tbsp) LEMON JUICE

300 ml (½ pt) SINGLE CREAM

Beat the egg yolks and sugar, and stir into the chestnut purée with the ginger, Cointreau and lemon juice. Stir in the cream. Chill and serve.

It will keep for 48 hours or so in the refrigerator.

LOVE POWDERS

*Recipes for love powders are mentioned constantly in literature from
the earliest times, in almost every civilization. Fascinating concoctions
of exotic and bizarre ingredients, their magical powers had great
importance. They were often dangerous, and many of them would not
be recommended today. For curiosity's sake, here are a few of them:*

"Take elecampane, the seeds and flowers, vervain and the
berries of mistletoe. Beat them, after being well dried in an
oven, into a powder, and give it to the party you design upon
in a glasse of wine and it will work wonderful effect to your
advantage."

This love powder, in Albertus Magnus' *Golden Cabinet of
Secrets*, is definitely not to be tried today. Although mistletoe
leaves are used in herbal remedies, the berries are poisonous.

Samuel Rowlands, in one of his Restoration plays, speaks
of a strange powder, which sounds rather less alarming:

> . . . *"Take me a turtle dove,*
> *and in an oven let her lie and bake*
> *So dry that you may powder of her make*
> *Which, being put into a cup of wine,*
> *The wench that drink'st it will to love incline."*

Even as late as the 18th century love powders were still
popular if John Gay, in *The Beggar's Opera*, is to be believed.
He wrote:

> *"Straight to the 'pothecary's shop I went*
> *and in love powder all my money spent."*

In the Far East love powders were widely used. Sir Richard
Burton, the Victorian traveller and translator of the *Kama
Sutra* and the *Arabian Nights*, gave us many of them. In the
Arabian Nights:

> *"The skin of a skink (lizard) reduced to powder and drunk*
> *with sweet white wine is a miraculous aphrodisiac."*

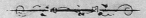

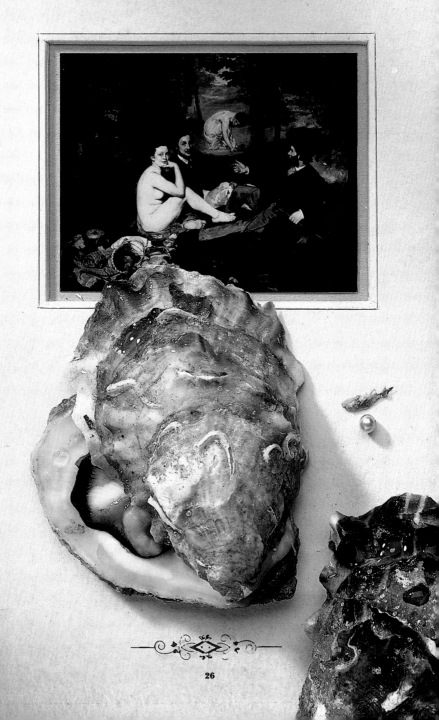

THE FOODS OF LOVE

In this chapter food in its many forms is discussed in detail – fish, meat, exotic spices, herbs, fruit, vegetables and plenty more. Although the ingredients come from all over the world – and in particular from the East with its long tradition of aphrodisiacs – they all have one thing in common: they are all reputed to enhance your love life, and in particular to help your libido to blossom. They range from quite ordinary food that you may already have in your larder or refrigerator – honey, chocolate, nuts, peaches and shellfish, for example – to the rare and exotic, including unusual Chinese herbs and oriental spices. Where appropriate, recipes have been included in each of the sections, but there are many more you can experiment with from your own cookery books, once you know the magical properties of the ingredients.

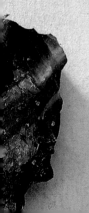

On the Seductive and Sensual Properties of

SEAFOOD AND FISH

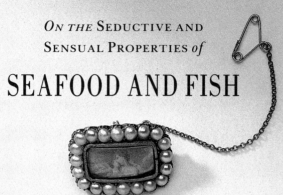

THE SEA IS ONE of the major sources of life. It is therefore no surprise that most sea creatures have the elements to form an aphrodisiac.

All shellfish, the strongest aphrodisiacs, contain phosphorus, calcium, iodine, iron, vitamin B and glyco-phosphates, basic essentials for an aphrodisiac. (An unfortunate few are allergic to shellfish, or some forms of it, so beware feasting on previously untasted types.) All oily fish, such as salmon, tuna, shark, eel, herring, mackerel and sardines, and many forms of white fish, including sole and turbot, contain phosphorus, calcium and vitamins A, B and D, basic essentials for a variety of aphrodisiac treats.

OYSTERS

The oyster is the *sine qua non* of aphrodisiacs. Connoisseurs eat oysters raw with their own juice, plus a little lemon juice, on a plate of crushed ice. They are so good eaten plain, when they really are at their most potent, that only the simplest and best recipes are worth considering.

LOBSTER

Most people eat only the white meat, but this is a grave mistake because according to the *cognoscenti*, the creamy substance and the green liver, as well as the coral roe in the hen lobsters, are also potent. Lobsters need no added aphrodisiacs. You can do no better than simply cook a lobster and serve it with a bottle of Chablis to make an exciting preamble to lovemaking.

CRAB

These are not quite as potent as lobsters, but they are much cheaper. Crab does need some preparation. A good way of serving it is to collect the crab meat, including the white from the claws, and put it in a food mill with canned red peppers, tomatoes, garlic, bouquet garni, lemon juice, gelatine, mayonnaise, cream and a tablespoon of nuoc nam (see page 69). Put a king prawn, followed by a layer of shrimps, into each of two greased moulds, then fill the moulds with the crab mixture. Chill before turning out the moulds; the king prawns should come out on top.

CLAMS

Americans have massive confidence in the aphrodisiac power of clams and American drillers brought the clam mania to the oil rigs in the North Sea. American quahogs started breeding in the United Kingdom in the 1920s after they were thrown uneaten and uncooked into the harbour from the liners' kitchens at the end of a voyage.

European clams, the Carpet and Venus for example, are eaten raw, like oysters.

WINKLES

Eaten voraciously by Stone Age people, as evidenced by the piles of shells at Skara Brae in Orkney, winkles were also popular with the North American Indians. In Belgium these

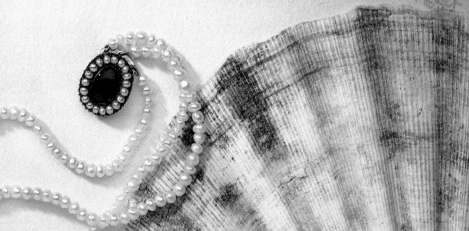

tiny aphrodisiacs are served with a mustard sauce on brown bread, in France with Chinese Nanja sauce in ramekins, and in England from a paper bag with vinegar.

COCKLES

Delicious cockles, a quiet little aphrodisiac, can be eaten raw or cooked. Chinese fish sauce transforms them into something else for the "dancing" bars of the Far East, which import quite a lot from Ireland, where they are plentiful.

MUSSELS

Throughout history the mussel, the peasant aphrodisiac of all Europe, has been carnival food. In medieval times, the word "*mossel*" also meant vulva. It was a medieval belief that witches could sail around the world in mussel shells, and at the Carnival of Ghent in 1538 the Queen of Fools always gave the King a carp and a bucket of mussels.

SCALLOPS

The scallop is a frisky aphrodisiac when cooked the right way. Its shell was the emblem of the Pilgrims, who followed their various routes to St Jacques de Compostela, and one scallop recipe is named after St Jacques. Eaten in all European countries, the many varieties vary in size from the 15 cm (6 in) Great Scallop, through Bay Scallops of 8cm (3 in), to 6 cm (2 in) Queens.

Scallops can be cooked in many ways – meunière, battered and deep fried, threaded on skewers and grilled or cooked carefully with dozens of herbs and wrapped in foil – all of them equally delicious.

EEL

This has the most powerful effect of all. The eel is born at sea, and after spending its life in rivers and lakes returns to the sea to spawn and die.

The French and Scandinavians buy their eels alive if possible, the Belgians smoke them and the English prefer to jelly them. The Egyptians ranked eels as gods and the Romans kept them in grand ponds and fed them special food. Eels eaten in Venice always seem to taste better than anywhere else. Smoked eel is a sophisticated aphrodisiac and makes an excellent *hors d'oeuvre*.

LAMPREY

Found both in the Atlantic and the Mediterranean, the lamprey is prized as an aphrodisiac. Medium-sized ones are best, and the French recipe for Lamprey à la Bordelaise with bacon and leek is splendidly sensual.

MACKEREL

The meaty flesh of mackerel, particularly when smoked, is popular all over Europe for making pâtés, providing a quick-acting aphrodisiac.

WHELKS

These can grow into a large marine snail, but are best eaten when small before their aphrodisiac powers are dissipated. Keep whelks in water for an hour, then boil them in their shells in salt water for 45 minutes and eat with a little vinegar, like winkles. Or boil them for 1½ hours, take them out and fry them with breadcrumbs, as the Greeks did, or just poach them, shelled, for 5 minutes, as the French do.

Dipping whelks in Nanja sauce helps to keep the aphrodisiac element up.

SHRIMPS AND PRAWNS

Prawns vary considerably in size, but the flavour and the aphrodisiacal element is much the same. The largest, Dublin Bay prawns (up to 24cm/9 in), are so called because they used to be sold there although they are actually fished many miles away.

The Japanese sometimes eat prawns live, as Europeans eat oysters. The living prawn is beheaded, shelled, gutted and put in the mouth while it is still wriggling.

ANCHOVIES

These have had a reputation as an aphrodisiac since the Ancient Greeks and in Provence, where the Ancient Greeks had their summer villas, they have been served with almost everything ever since. Six inches long, green when fresh, blue later, and black when ancient, they are good marinaded in white wine. The phosphorus in the wine, added to the aphrodisiac properties of the fish itself, gives a particular sparkle to the dish.

ANGEL FISH

As ugly as sin, this fish is surprisingly delicate in flavour. It has acquired a name as an aphrodisiac from medieval times, and is cooked in the same way as ray or skate.

CARP

This fish, with its golden scales, and huge reputation, has magic. Cooked Cantonese style , it is an aphrodisiac of quality. Carp was unknown to the Greeks and Romans, but familiar to the Renaissance; François I hand-fed his at Amboise, and his chefs made much of them, as his numerous progeny attest.

SALMON

The flesh of a wild salmon is pink from the red micro-organisms that form part of its diet. Hatchery-bred salmon are fed on paprika to make them look pink, a form of deceit. Neither of these fish has as much gusto in them as the wild salmon gains from its round trip of about 5,000 miles in the oceans. It is stronger than steak as an aphrodisiac and quicker acting by far.

SALMON TROUT

With the same diet as wild salmon and tasting similar, salmon trout has the same properties as an aphrodisiac. Norwegians have been fermenting trout for hundreds of years to preserve them, but also because it increases their aphrodisiacal strength. The Norwegian version is Rako Rret, strong, smelly and positive. Sur Stromming is the Swedish counterpart.

SHARK

These fish are found on both sides of the Atlantic from the Carolinas to Newfoundland, and from the Mediterranean to

Iceland. Shark steaks are considered an aphrodisiac, and are usually grilled and served with lemon juice. Shark fin has long been a favourite aphrodisiac of the discerning Chinese.

SWORDFISH

An oceanic fish, taken by harpoon, it is highly rated as an aphrodisiac by seamen. Serve it in 5cm (2 in) thick steaks, marinaded in lemon juice and grilled.

HERRING

An outstanding Irish way with herrings is to take a smoked fish, cut off its head, split it lengthwise, spread it in a dish, pour Irish whiskey over it and set it alight. It is ready when the flames die out, and should be eaten with home-made bread and a glass of Guinness. The Irish swear by this meal as *the* aphrodisiac.

KIPPER

The most aphrodisiacal of fish according to the people of Northumbria, where they were first invented by John Woodger of Seahouses in 1840. The best oak-smoked kippers come from Craster and Loch Fyne. They should be put in a jug of boiling water, head down, for ten minutes and served with brown bread and butter and poached eggs. Some say that they are more restorative of strength than inspiring.

TUNA

A magnificent fish up to 4m (13 ft) in length, with the wild strength of a Spanish bull, it is sadly uninspiring when tinned, when its potential is diminished by at least 70 per cent, Eaten fresh, it is an aphrodisiac of real consequence.

WHITE FISH

Sole, turbot, halibut, brill and huss all contain phosphorus, iodine and vitamins, which are good basic ingredients for an aphrodisiac.

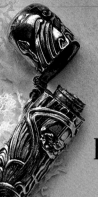

On the Seductive and
Sensual Properties *of*

CAVIAR AND
BOUILLABAISSE

B OTH THREE-STAR APHRODISIACS, these are renowned for
their power to awaken dormant desire, but they are
poles apart. Caviar, once eaten with golden spoons from
dishes of mother of pearl by the Tsars, is now consumed by
anyone who can afford it. Bouillabaisse was enjoyed originally by Venus as a pick-me-up after her demanding affairs
with Mars, and then by the Marseillais fishermen to whom
she gave the divine recipe in the second century BC, according
to legend.

BOUILLABAISSE

The Marseillais have kept it, unaltered and magical, ever
since. Lifelong friendships can end, however, over arguments
about the true constituents of this famous fish soup.

> *"A man who would put lobster in would poison wells.*
> *A man who would leave it out would starve his children."*
> (WAVERLEY ROOT, *The Food of France*)

The Marseillais, blessed with a really wide variety of fish, put
them all in, but especially *rascasse*, which lives in deep caves.
Langoustes (crayfish), crabs and sea spiders are essential,
while mussels and clams are inadmissible (although Parisians
use them). The crucial condiments and seasonings are olive
oil, saffron, onion, garlic, fennel, parsley, bay leaf, tomatoes
and orange peel.

The real aphrodisiac which starts this orchestra of seafood
off is the *rouille* that accompanies the soup. This is made of
garlic, black pepper, paprika and cayenne, mixed with bread-

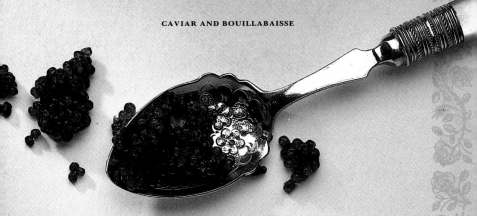

crumbs (or cooked potato) and olive oil. The mixture is spooned into the middle of the soup. Without it, the soup tastes sullen and lifeless.

Actually many provinces in France have their own bouillabaisse recipes – *cotriade* in Brittany, *chaudrée* in Poitou, *ttoron* in the Basque country and *pauchouse* in Burgundy. They all have something which brings out gusto in men and verve in women, but the undisputed king of them all is the Marseillaise bouillabaisse.

CAVIAR

In Russia caviar is called *ikra*. As an aphrodisiac, it is in the same class as oysters – easy to eat and digest. Excellent as an *hors d'oeuvre*, it is quick in action and a fine companion to champagne.

Real caviar is made from the ripe eggs of sturgeon, a fish found only in Northern waters, which feeds on phosphorus-based nutrients from the sea bed. There are more than 20 species. The largest is Beluga (James Bond's favourite) which can weigh up to 1600 kg (4,000 lb). Other species, *sevruga*, *osciotre* and *cipenser sturio*, weigh 10 to 20 kg (22-44 lb); the *sterylad* is the smallest at 5 kg (11 lb), and has the best caviar, which was always reserved for the Tsars and the emperors of the Austro-Hungarian Empire.

An elegant snack (if only orchids were more plentiful) would be lightly toasted bread covered with caviar, and layered with orchid petals.

ON THE SEDUCTIVE AND
SENSUAL PROPERTIES *of*

GAME

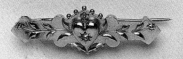

T HERE HAS ALWAYS been a mystique about hunting and
game in which the killing and eating of animals is
equated with the transfer of virility. It probably started with
Ashurbanipal, the Assyrian hunting king, whose stone lions
are now treasures in the British Museum. Arabian princes
and oil magnates, they say, by-pass hunting and simply eat
lions' testicles.

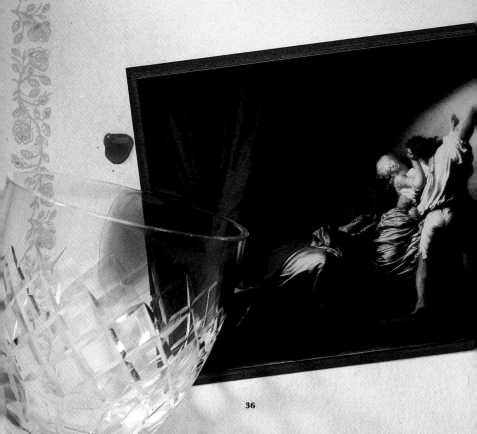

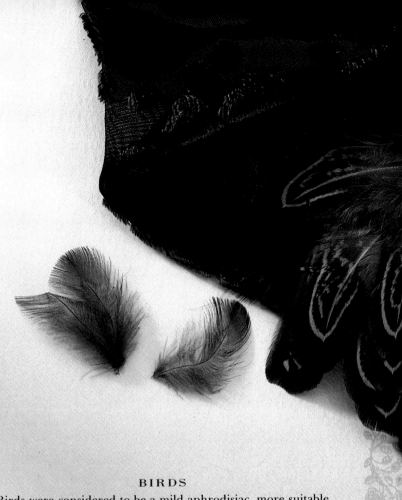

BIRDS

Birds were considered to be a mild aphrodisiac, more suitable for women; the men, perpetually macho, preferred wild boars and the testicles of stags. Henry IV of Navarre believed in the warm beatitude which partridge seems to produce in women and he even used to call on his mistress, Gabrielle d'Estrées, at her Paris house, 12 Rue Git Le Coeur, followed by a second coach in which was a chef with many cooked partridges, all kept hot in special dishes, with wine, sweetmeats and Armagnac besides. One evening Gabrielle was not at her best, and very tense (which completely destroys any hope of love or sensuality). Henry wondered what was wrong and then heard deep breathing from under the sofa, so he considerately handed down a partridge. This sort of thing was the beginning of the "intimate suppers" of the 18th and 19th centuries in private suites in hotels.

HARES

The hare has a special affinity with women and goddesses. Queen Boadicea carried one into battle. In mythology it is connected with the moon in India, China, Japan, Africa, North America and Europe. It was divine in the 21st Dynasty in Egypt and was Michabo, the Great Hare, creator of sun, moon and earth to the Algonquin Indians. In Britain it was sacred to the Earth mother in her day, so was not eaten. As one of Aphrodite's companions it appears with cupids on several Greek vases, and wedding rings bore the shape of a hare in Ancient Greece. It was also the favourite attendant of Eastre, the Anglo-Saxon goddess of dawn and fecundity, who gave us the pagan ancestry of some Easter customs. The Easter Hare, transmogrified into banal greetings cards, was the spring sacrifice. This creature's connections with magic, carnal love and fertility are impressive. Eat it if you dare.

Curnonsky, the ultimate connoisseur of cuisine in the Paris of the 1890s said,

> *"The hare is the prince of aphrodisiacs.*
> *If you know how to cook him."*

STAGS

Sir James Frazer, in *The Golden Bough* (1890), tells us that Renaissance stag hunts in France stemmed in part from the myth that the killing of a stag was linked with sexual potency, ensuring continued success in coition. (Perhaps this is why there is a collection of 2000 stags' antlers at the Château de Cheverny.)

Venison, well cooked, backs this theory up.

> *"There was a hunt of love too,*
> *with triumphant consummation.*
> *The hunt was a prelude to the*
> *pursuit of love, more tender,*
> *equally carnal."*
> MOLIÈRE

LA BOISETTE DE CHEVREUIL ST HUBERT

450 g (1 lb) SADDLE VENISON, BONED

15 ml (1 tbsp) FLOUR

50 g (2 OZ) UNSALTED BUTTER

30 ml (2 tbsp) COGNAC

300 ml (½ pt) GAME STOCK

60 ml (4 tbsp) RED WINE

60 ml (4 tbsp) DOUBLE CREAM

30 ml (2 tbsp) BLUEBERRY JELLY

MARINADE:

150 ml (¼ pt) RED WINE

½ ONION, CHOPPED

½ CARROT, CHOPPED

5 ml (1 tsp) CHOPPED PARSLEY

1 BAY LEAF

4 CLOVES

SPRIG OF ROSEMARY

4 JUNIPER BERRIES

Combine the ingredients for the marinade. Cut the venison into 2 pieces and leave it in the marinade in a cool place for 24 hours. Remove the venison, pat it dry, roll it in the flour and sauté in 60 ml (4 tbsp) butter until tender. Arrange on a hot serving dish and keep warm. Deglaze the pan with the cognac, add the game stock and wine and simmer for 5 minutes. Beat in the rest of the butter, add the cream and beat again. Reheat the sauce, but do not boil it. Spoon the sauce over the venison and serve with the blueberry jelly.

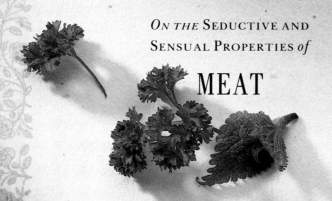

On the Seductive and Sensual Properties of

MEAT

IN THE LAST fifty years, foods for love have been changing radically, together with everything else, including both attitudes to love and how to perform the act of love.

STEAKS

In the 1930s it was thought that men needed rare steaks both to arouse desire and to keep up their stamina. (Havelock Ellis, the author of *Studies in the Psychology of Sex* [1897–1928] had recommended it as *the* male aphrodisiac.) Chateaubriand and Tournedos, Béarnaise and Rossini were the speedy means of achieving peaks of masculine vigour, compared with the long-drawn-out five-course meals that their fathers and grandfathers had enjoyed, with sherry before the meal, claret with it, port to follow, and often sleep as a finale.

The steaks of the '30s to '50s were not short cuts to peak performance, but Japanese steaks are just that. The Japanese can make best fillet steak go a long way, by freezing it and cutting it into thin slices, then refrigerating it and cutting it into thinner strips. These, along with the Chinese stir-fry steak dishes, are digested faster and taste better than a great chunk of rare steak.

One of the best Japanese steak dishes is the venerable Firepot or Steamboat (Shabu-Shabu), so-called because it is cooked at the table. There is also a similar Korean recipe, Gogi Bokum, using one pound of steak for four people, and with Bulgogi sauce, now available in Chinese food shops.

For an occasion requiring a lyrical consummation of

love, why not try Steak Tartare, preceded by oysters and followed by lychees, with not more than two glasses of wine and maybe an Armagnac afterwards.

SMOKED MEAT

The Europeans do have some similarly subtle meats, although they are not always to be found in the supermarkets. *Bunderfleisch*, for example, made in the Swiss mountains, with a secret formula using mountain herbs and white wine, creates surprisingly sudden strength, and pastrami can do the same, even when eaten standing up in a New York deli. Hams are also good for providing instant energy. Parma ham, for example, is delicious with green figs. *Lachsschinken* (called *Filet de Saxe* in France) with Roquefort cheese was often eaten by Casanova before his famous conquests.

Walking in the Dolomites you may be lucky enough to find and eat *bresaola* (dried beef fillet) which has been matured and marinated. Back in America, in the Kentucky mountains, you can find one of the best meats in the world – Kentucky ham (produced from hogs fed on clover, acorns, beans and grain), smoked over apple and hickory wood for 30 days, then "aged" for 12 months.

LAMB

The Japanese are not alone in finding enticing ways of cooking red meat. The Arabs have a deeper understanding of love and sex than most, and they have a particularly delicious

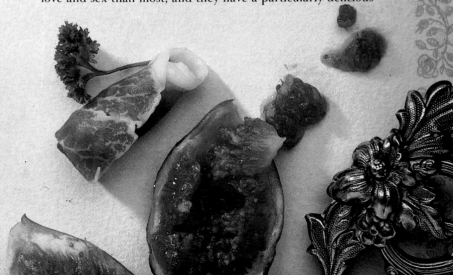

way of using herbs with lamb. An easily digested, quietly aromatic dish, eaten from shallow bowls, with yogurt, it is perfect as a preliminary to love-making.

Although the English have been eating lamb for centuries, this Arabian dish is more seductive than traditional roasts, especially when followed by fresh dates, sheeps' eyes (suitably enough), nougat and Turkish Delight, but with no wine at all, so as not to upset Allah.

ARABIAN LAMB

As this reheats well, it is worth making a larger quantity and freezing the remainder.

Serves 4

700 g (1½ lb) BONED LAMB SHOULDER, CUT INTO 2 cm (1 in) CUBES

30 ml (2 tbsp) OLIVE OIL

150 ml (¼ pt) WATER

1 CLOVE GARLIC, CHOPPED

2 ml (½ tsp) HERB-SALT

75 g (3 oz) BROWN LENTILS

2 CELERY STALKS, CHOPPED

2 CLOVES GARLIC

1 ml (¼ tsp) THYME

1 ml (¼ tsp) ROSEMARY

300 ml (½ pt) STOCK

TO GARNISH: FRESH MINT

Fry the lamb in the olive oil until brown and add the water, garlic and herb-salt. Place it in a heavy pan with more water and simmer until tender.

Cook the lentils, celery, garlic and herbs in the stock until the lentils are soft, but not disintegrating.

Mix the lamb and lentils together and keep warm over a low heat for half-an-hour.

Serve in shallow bowls, garnished with mint, with yogurt.

OYSTER BEEF SLICES

This dish is simple, easy to prepare, satisfying and quite potent for both sexes.

350 g (¾ lb) FILLET OR RUMP STEAK

5 ml (1 tsp) CORNFLOUR

5 ml (1 tsp) BROWN SUGAR

7.5 ml (1½ tsp) SOY SAUCE

45 ml (3 tbsp) MARROW BONE JELLY

15 ml (1 tbsp) SHERRY

10 ml (2 tsp) SUNFLOWER OIL

2 SPRING ONIONS, CUT INTO 4 cm (2 in) PIECES

10 ml (2 tsp) OYSTER SAUCE

Cut the beef into thin slices. Dredge with the cornflour and sugar. Add the soy sauce, marrow bone jelly and sherry, and toss. Leave for 15 minutes. Heat the oil in a wok over a high heat. Stir-fry the beef slices for 1 minute. Add the spring onions and stir-fry for another minute. Then add the oyster sauce, stir and serve.

CARPET BAG STEAK

The combination of steak and oysters is a sure-fire winner.

2 THICK FILLET STEAKS

8 OYSTERS

25 g (1 oz) MUSHROOMS

SALT AND PEPPER

10 ml (2 tsp) OLIVE OIL

Cut the steaks almost through horizontally, open them out and spread 4 oysters and half the mushrooms on one cut surface of each steak. Fold over and sew up with a trussing needle and fine string. Brush the steaks with oil and cook under a hot grill for 5 minutes each side or according to taste. Remove the string before serving.

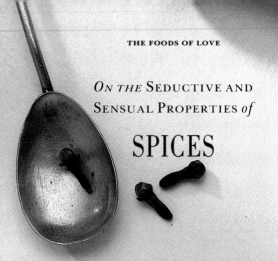

On the Seductive and Sensual Properties *of*

SPICES

T HE SPICE TRADE is one of the oldest known to man, the spices themselves used in religious rites and medicine, and as aphrodisiacs, long before their culinary use became popular. Arabs carefully withheld the true source of spices, and spread fantastic tales about them: that they grew in lakes guarded by winged beasts, and in forests infested by poisonous snakes, which added to their mystique.

The immense annual income of King Solomon, for example, came from the *"traffic of the spice merchants"* (Kings, 10:15). This was at a time when spices were used for their effective power during religious rites and as aphrodisiacs for the rich and powerful.

Richard Burton's translation of the *Arabian Nights* included several love potions involving a splendid mixture of many different spices.

DURAN SEEDS

These come from a tree that grows in India and Malaya. The large seeds taste like almonds and are ground up to make a powerful aphrodisiac.

DITA BARK

This comes from a tree growing in Australia and India. It is suggested in the *Ananga Ranga* that the seeds are an aphrodisiac if kept in the mouth during sexual union.

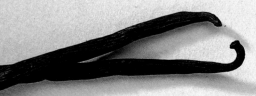

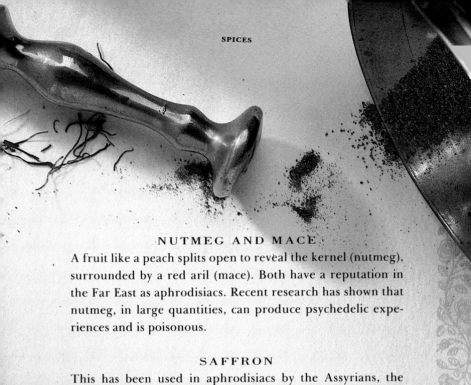

NUTMEG AND MACE

A fruit like a peach splits open to reveal the kernel (nutmeg), surrounded by a red aril (mace). Both have a reputation in the Far East as aphrodisiacs. Recent research has shown that nutmeg, in large quantities, can produce psychedelic experiences and is poisonous.

SAFFRON

This has been used in aphrodisiacs by the Assyrians, the Phoenicians, the Greeks (who believed that if a girl took saffron for a week she could not resist a lover), the Arabs and even the British, who grew it at Saffron Walden from the mid-14th century. It is extremely expensive because it takes 100,000 saffron crocus flowers to produce 450 g (1 lb) of saffron. It is claimed that saffron stimulates the uterus and promotes blood circulation.

VANILLA

Yellow flowers are followed by long aromatic pods which when dried form vanilla beans. Used by the Aztecs to improve their chocolate and by the French in their early chocolate making, it is now commonly used in ice cream. Mildly aphrodisiac.

> *"Madeira wine with ginger,*
> *cinnamon, rhubarb and vanilla*
> *makes a wine with aphrodisiac properties."*
>
> CULPEPER, *The Complete Herbal*

TABASCO PEPPER/CAYENNE

The tropical white-petalled, yellow-centred flowers produce oblong pods that contain red and yellow seeds, which, when pulverized, make this pepper. In Georgian times special silver pots with long thin spoons were made for it. Young bloods used it as an aphrodisiac – it stimulates blood circulation – and old men took it to cure cramp. As a revitalizer, try one teaspoon of cayenne pepper in a small glass of tomato juice.

SICHUAN PEPPER

Known as "flower pepper" in China, this is a pleasant and noticeably effective spice, going straight to the solar plexus. In China it is used as part of an aphrodisiac mixture, with ginseng and ginger in equal parts.

CINNAMON

Both the dried inner bark of the tropical evergreen tree and coarsely ground seed are used. The bark is an antiseptic, astringent and stimulant as well as an aphrodisiac.

"Green peas boiled with onions,
together with cinnamon, ginger and
cardamoms, all ground, create
passion and strength in coitus."
THE PERFUMED GARDEN

CARDAMOM

Whole cardamom seeds are used for flavouring marinades and curries. They are mentioned in a *Kama Sutra* recipe as an aphrodisiac, *"mixed with ginger and cinnamon, spread over onions and peas"*.

CLOVES

The little spikes are unopened flower buds, which have been sun dried, and form part of several aphrodisiac potions.

STAR ANISE

This is an Asiatic spice made from the grey-brown fruits of the bush, *Illicium verum*, which dry into eight-pointed stars tasting of liquorice. Use sparingly, in drinks as well as food.

BLACK PEPPER

Tropical white flowers are followed by the aromatic, wrinkled fruits, which must be used freshly ground. Attila the Hun demanded 3,000 lb of pepper as part of the ransom *"not to sack Rome"*. It is a tonic, stimulative and carminative.

"Make a compound of pepper,
lavender, galaga, musk, honey and
ginger. Wash the member in warm
water, and anoint it with the mixture".

THE PERFUMED GARDEN

CHILLIES

The name is Aztec, whose people used them for 5,000 years, but chillies have been grown and used worldwide since Columbus. There are innumerable varieties.

GINGER

An aphrodisiac in use in China for 3,000 years, and in Europe since the Middle Ages. The creeping rhizomes provide the spice. Dried ginger powder is more pungent, but most Chinese recipes insist on young, peeled root, as it stimulates circulation.

"Men who suddenly do not feel
strong enough to enjoy women,
should eat ginger, honey, byrether,
hellebore, garlic, cinnamon, cloves,
nutmeg, cardamoms, sparrow's
tongues (a herb) and long pepper
immediately."

THE PERFUMED GARDEN

JUNIPER

The blue berries come from an evergreen of the cypress family and take two years to ripen. Crushed or chopped fine, juniper berries are a natural companion to most game, creating an aphrodisiac of a special kind. According to the *Kama Sutra* juniper berries steeped in water make a *"drink for vigour"*. (Juniper berries should not be taken during pregnancy or if you have a liver condition.)

ON THE SEDUCTIVE AND SENSUAL PROPERTIES *of*

HERBS

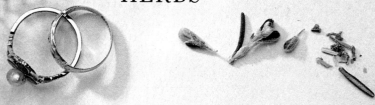

Hᴇʀʙꜱ ʜᴀᴠᴇ ʟᴏɴɢ had a reputation as aphrodisiacs, among their other medicinal properties.

MYRTLE

This was planted around the temples dedicated to Aphrodite in Greece, to commemorate the wreath she was wearing when Paris awarded her the Golden Apple for her beauty. (On a more practical note, she was also reputed to use myrtle in a vaginal douche.) In Roman times it was a traditional decoration at weddings, while distillation of two handfuls of myrtle flowers and leaves in two quarts of spring water with a quart of white wine *"beautifies, and when mixed with cordial syrup, inclines those that drink to be very amorous"*.

There was also the 18th-century Portuguese aphrodisiac known as Angel Water – too expensive to recreate nowadays because it contains ambergris. It consists of 600 ml (1 pt) of orange flower water, 600 ml (1 pt) of rose water, 300 ml (½ pt) myrtle water, 400 ml (14 fl oz) distilled spirit of musk and 400 ml (14 fl oz) spirit of ambergris, all shaken together like a cocktail.

WILD MARJORAM

Aphrodite's sweet breath is reputed to have created the scent of wild marjoram; it is another plant that is closely associated with her, *". . . fair Venus raised the plant, which from the Goddess' touch derived its scent"*.

It was also used to crown young couples in Rome, and symbolized happiness. In many parts of Europe, including

England, it is still possible to lie on a bank of wild marjoram, enjoying the bitter-sweet scent given off by the bruised leaves. The name for it, oregano (*oros* = mountain, *ganos* = joy), is very apt. John Gerard in his 16th-century herbal prescribed it to those "*given much to sighing*". Perhaps its purpose in love potions was to relax and warm the inhibited.

VER·VAIN

This herb is also sacred to Venus, and its magical powers have been recognized by the Egyptians, Chinese, Romans, Druids, Persians and Anglo-Saxons. Its Latin name is *Herba veneris*, because of the aphrodisiac powers attributed to it. It forms part of the "*true love powder*" in *The Golden Cabinet of Secrets* (see page 25).

ROSEMARY

This was worn at weddings and, in the 16th century, gilded twigs were offered to guests. In *The Queen's Delight* of 1695, it was said that, "*It comforteth the heart, the stomach, the brain and all the nervous parts of the body*". And its medicinal properties do indeed both calm palpitations and stimulate the brain and nervous system.

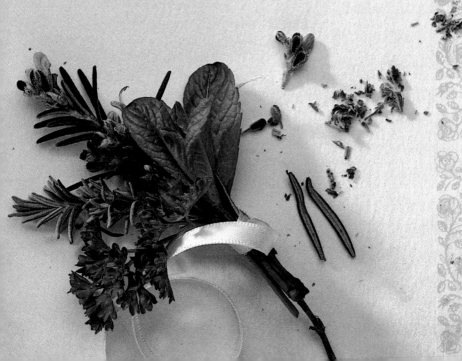

MEADOWSWEET

Another herb often strewn at weddings was meadowsweet (also called bridewort), *"for the smell thereof makes the heart merrie and joyful and delighteth the senses"*. Salicylic acid, the basic ingredient of aspirin, was first derived from it in the 19th century, thus justifying centuries of herbal lore. Although the wedding herbs are all edible, it is primarily for their fragrance that they are used on these occasions.

FENNEL

This and the following herb are perhaps more male oriented. Fennel, used by Roman warriors for strength, and by most cooks with fish, is also referred to in the *Kama Sutra*. *"If ghee, honey, sugar and liquorice in equal quantities, the juice of the fennel plant and milk are mixed together, the nectar is said to be holy, and provocative of sexual vigour."*

FENUGREEK

This contains diosgenin, used in the synthesis of sex hormones. The seeds contain phosphoric acid and, when roasted, have been used for centuries as an aphrodisiac. They are sold in Chinese health food shops as a restorative.

SEA HOLLY

Eryngo or sea holly, with its blue thistle-like flowers, grows wild in profusion on the sea coasts of Devon and Cornwall. It used to be sold in candied form, and was alluded to by Falstaff in *The Merry Wives of Windsor: "Hail kissing comfits, and snow eringoes"*. It was the roots which were called kissing comfits, a reference to their aphrodisiac properties. They are also mentioned in Dryden's translation of Juvenal's *Satires*,
> *"Who lewdly danced at a midnight ball*
> *For hot eryngoes and fat oysters call"*.

MINT

The Arabs have always believed that mint increases virility, and modern herbalists prescribe it for cases of impotence and decreased libido. No cooking is necessary. Peppermint is good added to bathwater, as it restores vigour.

CHINESE HERBS

The West has long been fascinated by the *Materia Medica* of China, with its promise of health, longevity, increased sexual potency, fertility and rejuvenation. The Emperor Shen Nung (the Divine Husband-man) gave China its healing medicines, as well as its agriculture, in the third millennium BC. Shen Nung also produced the first *Pen Ts'ao (Great Herbal)* in 2700 BC and the Chinese have been continuing the work ever since.

The herbs listed here are available from Chinese health food shops.

ACANTHOPANAX SPINOSUM Used as a tonic and anti-rheumatic, and for restoring vigour and sexual potency. Dose: 5–10 g

CALLOTARIA URSINA (male genitalia of the sealion) Used as a tonic in impotence and sterility. Dose 2–4 g

CORNUS OFFICINALIS Used as a tonic in impotence. Dose: 5–10 g

CUSCUTA JAPONICA Used as a tonic in impotence caused by prostate gland problems. Dose: 7–15 g

EPIMEDIUM MACRANTHUM Extract of leaves used as an aphrodisiac. Dose: 3–8 g

GYNOMORIUM COCCINEUM Used as a tonic and aphrodisiac. Has sperm-producing properties. Dose: 4–11 g

LIGUSTRUM JAPONICUM Used as a nutrient tonic. Dose 5–15 g

SELINUM MONNIERE Used as a stimulant; aphrodisiac. Dose: 5–10 g

HU-LU-FA (for men only) Used as a tonic to the reproductive system and generative organs. It contains amino acids, and vitamins A and D. It also contains trimethylamine, a sex hormone. Dose: 8–10 tablets a day

DONG QUAI TANG KWEI (for women only) Improves blood, nourishes female glands. Comes in bundles like asparagus or in powder form or capsules. Dose: As directed on the packet

TSAN-TS'AI Used to improve condition of all female organs and remove inflammation. Dosage is outlined on the packet.

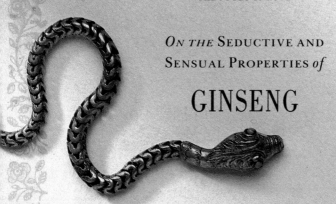

On the Seductive and Sensual Properties of

GINSENG

MEDICAL SCIENTISTS have always been cautious about aphrodisiacs, but since the 1960s, when experiments with humans in Russia and the United States confirmed its properties, they have put out reports saying that ginseng, taken on a regular basis, produces "a positive increase in physical and mental efficiency, sexual potency, and an overall sense of well-being".

Asian ginseng is derived from *Panax schinseng*, a plant of the *Araliaceae* family, found growing wild in Manchuria, Korea and Russia. A strengthener of the central nervous system and the spinal cord, ginseng is also a nutrient which maintains the balance of body and spirit. But it does not work instantly. It must be an everyday element of the diet for about three months before any effect is discernible. Keep to the recommended doses, because ginseng can be dangerous in large quantities, and continuous use over many months is not recommended.

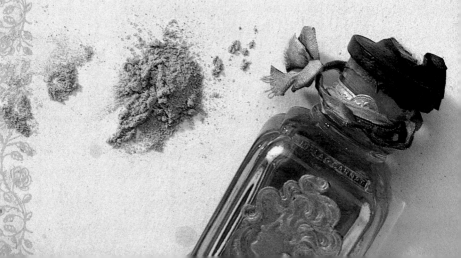

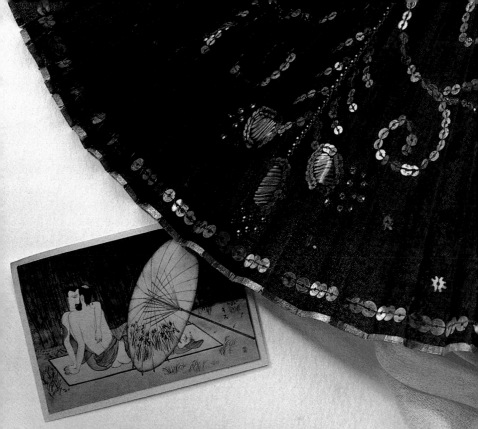

FORMS OF GINSENG

Various forms of ginseng are obtainable from Chinese health food shops, which will supply information on dosages:

JIN SAM JUNG This is a bottled extract consisting of Korean ginseng root (whole), ginseng extract, honey and royal jelly.

KOREAN GINSENG COMPLEX This is a blend of ginseng root powder, royal jelly, PABA (para-amino-benzoic acid) and vitamin E, the fertility vitamin.

CHINESE PROCESSED GINSENG COMPOUND This is super ginseng in the form of nuggets to make tea, containing 16 roots, with 42 minerals. (Do not take any vitamin C for 3 hours after drinking this compound.)

FO-TI-TIENG This is available as tea sachets or capsules. The best form is Chinese Instant Fo-Ti-Tieng, a tonic, detoxifier, and energy booster that relieves rheumatism, neuralgia and gout and has been used for centuries in China.

YUAN SHENG SHENG TI These are energy herbs which include juniper berries for virility and strength.

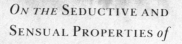

On the Seductive and Sensual Properties of

VEGETABLES

VEGETARIANS TAKE HEART. Vegetables prevail among the foods listed by Sir Richard Burton (1821–90) as *"lascivious meats"*; peas, broad beans, radishes, artichokes, lettuce, leeks and onions are all confirmed as having aphrodisiacal properties by earlier writers.

Johann Jakob Wecker (1570–1657) was also a great believer in vegetables, *"If any man desire to be a strong soldier in the camp of Venus, let him be armed with such meat; chiefly with bulbous roots for they all provoke venery"*. He also specifically mentions the onion, which is a member of the lily family, and is the flower bulb consumed most widely around the world. The Babylonians taught the Egyptians that the onion was the symbol of perfection, and they, in their turn, worshipped it to the extent of not eating it at all. The Greeks noticed that onions *"dim the eyes and excite amatory propensities"* but also that even the onion *"will do you no good if you have no strength yourself"*.

ROOT VEGETABLES

Carrots and parsnips were also well thought of by the ancients. Carrots were so commonplace in love philtres that the Greeks called the vegetable "philtron". The Elizabethans considered them to be *"a great furtherer of Venus, her pleasure, and love's delight"*. Parsnip is said by Orpheus to be an aphrodisiac, the wild variety being regarded as more potent than the cultivated form.

The humble potato was also reputed to have aphrodisiac powers in the 17th century, and is frequently mentioned in this context in Elizabethan drama.

ASPARAGUS

This has been cultivated since 200 BC as an aristocrat among vegetables, and still grows in its wild form along the sandy coasts of France, in Greece and profusely on the Russian Steppes. It *"manifestly provoketh Venus"*. The Romans had a saying, *"Do it quicker than you can cook asparagus"* – about 15 minutes. In the 16th century, Shaykh Umar Ibn Muhammed Al Nefzawi said, in *The Perfumed Garden*, that asparagus, *"with yolk of egg fried in fat, camels' milk and honey causes the virile member to be on the alert, night and day"*.

TRUFFLES

These are, literally, the earthiest aphrodisiac. The truffle is an edible fungus, indigenous to Europe, positively recommended as an aphrodisiac by Brillat-Savarin, the 19th-century French gourmet, used by Napoleon as such, and strongly advised by all French chefs for its special qualities in *haute cuisine*. However, the knowledgeable methods of cooking truffles used by Colette, described in *Earthly Paradise*, could become the basis of an exquisite weekend spent amidst the walnut groves of the Perigord. First she describes *"The true truffle, the black truffle, the truffle of Perigord . . ."* and goes on with detailed cooking instructions:

"bathed in a good very dry white wine . . . salted
without extravagance, peppered with discretion, they can
be cooked in a simple, black, cast-iron
stewpan with the lid on. For twenty-five minutes they
must dance in the constant flow of bubbles
drawing with them through the eddies and the
foam – like tritons playing round some darker Amphitrite
– a score or so of smallish strips of bacon fat, but
not too fat, which will give body to the stock. No other
herbs or spices. Do not eat the truffle without wine".

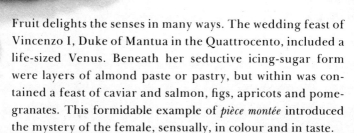

On the Seductive and Sensual Properties *of*

FRUIT

Fruit delights the senses in many ways. The wedding feast of Vincenzo I, Duke of Mantua in the Quattrocento, included a life-sized Venus. Beneath her seductive icing-sugar form were layers of almond paste or pastry, but within was contained a feast of caviar and salmon, figs, apricots and pomegranates. This formidable example of *pièce montée* introduced the mystery of the female, sensually, in colour and in taste.

The following is a selection of some of the best fruit.

FIGS

Like oysters, these need nothing but their own inimitable qualities. There is a richness of texture and a depth to the succulence of the flesh which makes all other fruits insipid.

Saturn first discovered the fig. In Ancient Greece, it had its most profane uses in the winter festival of Saturnalia. Eating blue-black figs, with their dark red seeds, is a quiet orgy in itself, which no grape, peach or mulberry can match for sheer sensual pleasure.

QUINCE

The pale golden quince was said to be the original apple which lured Eve, but to the Greeks and Romans this fragrant fruit was sacred to Venus, who is often shown with it in her hand (it was a gift from Paris to celebrate her beauty).

"The eating of a Quince pear at weddings is said to be preparative
of sweet and delightful dayes between the married persons."
JOHN CASE *The Praise of Musicke*

POMEGRANATES

Both from their shape and their startling vividness, pomegranates, when cut through, have been a symbol of fecundity
since Solomon entertained Sheba. The bride in the *Song of
Songs* said "*I would give you mulled wine to drink and the fresh
juice of pomegranates*". In a special aphrodisiac (see page 15),
the smooth skin and piquant flesh are ground to a powder
and mixed with ground almonds, pumpkin and sesame seeds
and honey. It has a taste like *halva,* but stronger, and later,
brings a strange sensation with it.

PEACHES

Among the many varieties of French peach there is one
known as *le sein de Venus* (Venus' breast). "*A big round fruit
with a nipple on the top, crimson flush, and rather fine semi-melting
flesh, quite good in flavour.*" Albertus Magnus, the medieval
herbalist, says that "*the peach increases intercourse*"; and the
Buch der Natur has it that "*for afflicted men that are impotent
because of a cold nature it is good to induce passion*"

BANANAS

The serpent that tempted Eve hid in a bunch of bananas,
hence the banana's Latin name of *Musa paradisica* (fruit of
paradise) or *Musa sapienta* (fruit of knowledge). If, as the
legend has it, Ceylon (now Sri Lanka) was the Garden of
Eden, Adam's original modesty was probably covered with a
banana leaf.

The word "banana" is itself African. In Central Africa
banana leaves are believed to be capable of fertilizing women,
and if a woman can prove that a flower has fallen on her
back, she is honourably acquitted of infidelity. Banana
blossom also appears in Filipino recipes as an aphrodisiac.

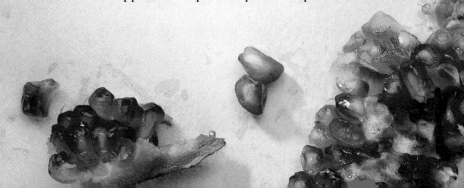

On the Seductive and Sensual Properties of

CHOCOLATE

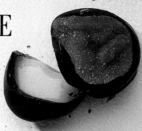

Made by the Peruvians Indians from the cacao bean, chocolate was offered to deities at births, weddings, puberty rites and funerals as well as to generals and to the bravest soldiers after battle. It was also the standard currency in Peru.

The Indians believed in the power of chocolate as an aphrodisiac. Montezuma, who maintained a harem of 600 odalisques, was said to drink 50 cups of it a day from a goblet of solid gold.

HISTORICAL USES

The first foreigners to receive cacao beans disregarded them. In 1502 Christopher Columbus gave some to King Ferdinand of Spain, who was not interested. Sir Francis Drake brought a ton of them back to England, taken from a Spanish galleon together with bars of silver, but the cacao beans were mistaken for sheep droppings and thrown into Plymouth harbour, thus robbing Queen Elizabeth I of an interesting experience. At some point they must have become accepted, as Casanova recommended chocolate as an aphrodisiac. Madame du Barry – Louis XV's mistress – gave it to her lovers, and the entourage of Louis XIV drank it several times a day. In England, in the 17th century, the royal physician, Henry Stubbs, declared that *"chocolate is provocative to lust"*.

Research chemists now admit that it is a mild aphrodisiac. Chocolate contains caffeine and theobromine, both of which stimulate the central nervous system, and phenylethylamine, which is similar to amphetamines and has an effect rather like the emotional highs and lows of being in love.

CHOCOLATE RECIPES

Alexander Dumas, in his *Grand Dictionnaire de Cuisine*, suggests making chocolate the night before and leaving it: *"The repose of the night concentrates it, and gives it a velvet quality. Then reheat it and serve in a porcelain coffee pot."* He recommends it as an aphrodisiac and as a pick-me-up after love-making:

> *"Well then, if any man has drunk too*
> *deeply from the cup of voluptuousness*
> *. . . let him take a good half litre of*
> *ambergris-flavoured chocolate in the*
> *proportions of 72 grains of ambergris to*
> *half a kilo of chocolate and marvels will*
> *be witnessed".*

Brillat-Savarin reiterates this statement in *Le Trésor Gastronomique de France*.

Crème de cacao, a chocolate liqueur, drunk with a dash of orange bitters and vodka, is a pleasant way to take this mild aphrodisiac.

CHOCOLATE NUT TRUFFLES

These are best eaten on a rug in front of a good fire.

100 g (4 OZ) MIXED NUTS, ROUGHLY CHOPPED

125 g (5 OZ) BITTER CHOCOLATE

25 g (1 OZ) UNSALTED BUTTER

50 g (2 OZ) ICING SUGAR

30 ml (2 tbsp) COCOA POWDER

Lightly roast the nuts. Melt the chocolate with the butter in a bowl over a pan of hot water and then blend with the nuts and sugar in a food processor. Chill the mixture and form into small balls. Roll them in cocoa powder.

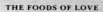

ON THE SEDUCTIVE AND
SENSUAL PROPERTIES *of*

NUTS

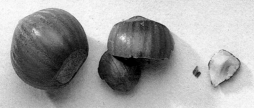

Nuts have long been highly regarded as an aphrodisiac and pistachios have been found in Jordan dating from 6760 bc. In King Solomon's garden walnuts, pistachios and almonds grew in profusion. The Greeks and Romans invariably used them in marriage ceremonies, throwing walnuts instead of rice, and burning hazel torches as a token of fertility and to ensure a happy marriage.

HAZELNUTS

Virgil praised the filbert above the vine, the myrtle and the bay tree for its aphrodisiac powers. Hazelnuts, according to the *Hortus Sanitatis*, when mixed with satyrion *"will enable a man to satisfy all the desires of his wife"*, and their value in curing male impotence was noted in *Physica in Patrologia Latina*.

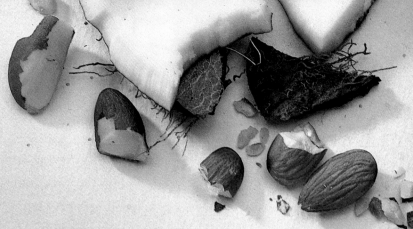

CHESTNUTS

According to the no-nonsense Elizabethans *"chestnuts, being flatulent, incite Venus"* and chestnuts are used in a love potion in J. J. Wecker's *Book of Secrets* . *"Take chestnuts steeped in Muscadet, then boil them with satyrions (10), land crocodiles (2), pine kernels (4 oz), pistachios (4 oz), rocket seed (2 oz), cubebs (1 oz), cinnamon (1/2 oz), sugar (12 oz)."*

COCONUT

In northern India, home of the *Kama Sutra* and the *Ananga Ranga*, the coconut is not only a symbol of fertility, but is kept by priests to give to women who wish to conceive.

WALNUTS

Used by the Romans in fertility rites, walnuts are still used today by some African tribes as a remedy for male sterility. A recipe for walnut cream is given in the Love Potions on page 18.

PISTACHIOS

The Queen of Sheba was said to have monopolized the supply of pistachios in Syria, for herself and her favourites, because they *"awaken desire"*.

ALMONDS

These are closely related to the peach and the apricot, and all are used in potions to improve sexual relations. It was the Crusaders in the 12th century who brought back a taste not only for spices but for creamy almond sauces and confections such as nougat and marzipan.

On the Seductive and Sensual Properties *of*

FLOWERS

"Roses, the garden's pride
Are flowers for love and flowers for kings,
In courts desired and weddings."

THOMAS CAMPION

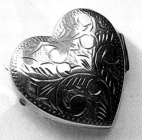
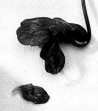

Almost any flowers enhance love. Their perfection of form and texture, and above all their fragrance, make them the simplest and most elegant expression of love. The cycle from bud through to bloom and from fertilization to fruit is a visually satisfying equivalent to human biology. And they produce nectar for honey, the most feminine of aphrodisiacs.

FLOWERS FOR WEDDINGS

The Saracens gave us the custom of carrying orange blossoms in bridal bouquets. The flowers symbolize chastity, and can be infused to make a mild nerve tonic. For a passionate wedding night the bride should wear a nosegay of violets and periwinkles, and nibble the flowers before climbing into bed with her bridegroom.

Roman brides and grooms were crowned with roses, as were images of Venus and Cupid. Nero demanded that his hosts fill their fountains with rose water, cover the ground with rose leaves and provide him with rose wine to drink and bathe in. Cleopatra waded ankle deep in rose petals.

VIOLETS

The violet, according to Culpeper, is *"a fine plant of Venus"*, who, as the goddess of bloom and beauty, protectress of gardens, cares for its most modest inhabitants. John Parkinson, botanist to Charles I, recommended the use of the dog violet – *"the roote hereof is held to be of more efficacy in venereous effects than any of the Orchids or Satyrions"*.

Violets and valerian are mentioned in Albertus Magnus' *Golden Cabinet of Secrets*, as having *"love-provoking powers"* if picked in the last quarter of the moon.

VIOLET SHERBET

60 ml (4 tbsp) CRÈME DE VIOLETTE

200 ml (⅓ pt) SUGAR SYRUP

300 ml (½ pt) GRAPE JUICE

30 ml (2 tbsp) LIME JUICE

1 EGG WHITE

50 g (2 OZ) CASTER SUGAR

Mix the liquid ingredients in a bowl, freeze until it reaches the mushy stage, then beat the egg white, fold in the caster

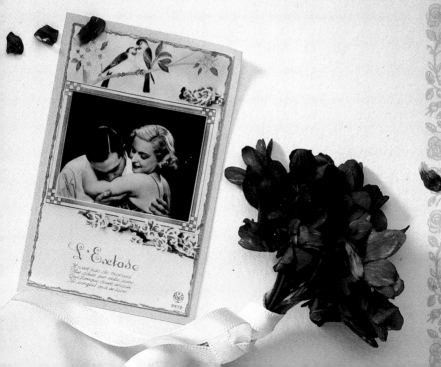

sugar, and add to the mixture. Refreeze. Serve in glasses decorated with violet blossoms.

ORCHIDS AND BULBS

Of all the parts of the flower it is the bulb that has the greatest claim to efficacy as a true aphrodisiac, in particular the orchid bulb. The wild orchid, known as satyrion, created the Greek and Roman aphrodisiac *in excelsis*, according to many sources. The root, it was said *"causeth great heat and therefore it giveth lust unto the works of generation"*. If you combine it with hazelnuts and wine, as directed in a recipe for a nightcap in the *Hortus Sanitatis "thou wilt that night be potent and give pleasure to thy wife"*. In the same volume, you will find advice on how to choose the sex of the ensuing child, by eating either the "larger" or "lesser" part of the bulb.

Over-use of the orchid caused it to become an endangered species, particularly from too much of the very popular "Salop" being drunk in the 18th century. Now it is as unusable as rhinoceros horn, for reasons of scarcity, although obviously it had a far greater claim in the first place as a genuine aphrodisiac. A cheap and relatively available substitute is the tuber of the cyclamen, which is purported to have some effect.

For those who seek "the door of love", try gladiolus and asphodel bulbs, sliced and sprinkled with cumin and pounded and boiled in water, formed into flat cakes, fried in oil and served with thyme, pepper, oregano and honey. In *The Assembly Women* by Aristophanes, the old hag says to the reluctant young man, *"Oh, you'll manage all right; all you need is a plateful of tulip bulbs"*.

ROYAL JELLY AND HONEY

Flowers also provide the initial source of two of the best-known aphrodisiacs, royal jelly and honey.

A colony of bees consists of one queen, several hundred drones, and between 25,000 and 100,000 workers and provides these valuable aphrodisiacs. The queen is fed exclusively on royal jelly, a whitish solution secreted by the glands of female worker bees. Royal jelly contains all the amino acids, together with ten vitamins and six minerals, but it is not cheap. Variations in price of shop-bought royal jelly relate to the additional ingredients in the product, and their quantities. Ginseng, serenoa and damiana are all found as additives. Royal jelly and ginseng, both life enhancing, have been used in China and the East for centuries and are becoming increassingly popular in the West.

Honey is used in many aphrodisiac mixtures. Ottaviano Bon, the 17th-century Venetian diplomat who visited the Seraglio in Top Kapi, tells us, *"The honeys which are consumed by the seraglio are in enormous amounts, because they are used in all food, as well as in sherbets for poorer folk, and come from Walachia, Transylvania and Moldavia"*.

Honey extracted from poisonous plants can itself be poisonous, so, by the same token, bees that have gathered nectar from flowers which are aphrodisiac, like jasmine, do make aphrodisiacal honey. This may explain the reputation as an aphrodisiac of the Greek Hymettus honey, flavoured as it is with wild marjoram and myrtle (both favourites of Aphrodite). Honey is also one of the most easily assimilated sources of energy, quickly giving a boost to blood sugar levels. Carefully selected honey is therefore an essential item in a lover's store cupboard.

Just as honey is at the heart of flower and fruit production, it is also a constant in the preparation of aphrodisiacs. In *The Perfumed Garden*, the 16th-century book by Shayk Umar Ibn Muhammed Al Nefzawi, we are exhorted to *"Anoint the member with the blood of a he-goat mixed with honey, for a night of real splendour"*.

On the Seductive and
Sensual Properties of

STRANGE APHRODISIACS

THE VERY NATURE of aphrodisiacs presupposes something unusual. Their function, to enhance the pleasure
of sexual intercourse or to create desire where none exists,
suggests some kind of magic. Certainly some aphrodisiacs
come from strange sources, including some of the following.

AMBERGRIS
This is a wax-like substance, found floating in tropical seas,
and also in the intestines of the sperm whale. It has had a
reputation as an aphrodisiac since the time of the Ancient
Greeks. It is difficult to obtain and immensely expensive,
although only three grains are required for most recipes.

HIPPOMANES
This is one of the sure-fire aphrodisiacs, described in the
Oxford Dictionary as *"a small black fleshy substance said to occur
on the forehead of a new-born foal; also a mucous humour
that runs from mares a-horsing. Both reputed aphrodisiacs"*. Originally it was Tibullus, the Roman poet, who said that it was
fluid from mares in heat, and Virgil who described it as the
membrane on the forehead of a newborn colt, bitten off and
eaten by the mare. Pliny the Elder said of it,

> *"If a person can remove this before
> the mare, he has a powerful philtre
> to engender passion. The mere odour
> of it will make any animal frantic
> and humans also, especially
> women."*

CAMEL'S MILK

This was mentioned repeatedly in Arabian potions, in which it was mixed with honey and dates. It is normally available, dried, in Chinese health food shops; take 15 mg per kilogram of your weight.

BOISS BANDE

This is an aphrodisiac made in the West Indies, with a strong reputation there. It consists of the bark of a tree (which contains bucin and strychnine) tied up and boiled in water which is then drunk, hence the name. It is not recommended, as it is dangerous if taken to excess.

BULLS' BLOOD

Obtained from bulls' testes, and coagulated by boiling or baking, this is sold in the markets near the bullrings, to be put into *sangre con pimentos*, *sangre con cebolla* and *fritos mallorquine*. These are bullfighters' snacks and all carry strong reputations as aphrodisiacs in Spain. (They are efficient – I can recommend them.)

COCKS' COMBS

Catherine de Medici's favourite meal consisted of cocks' combs, but it did her no good, as Henry II spent all his time and energy with Diane de Poitier. Other parts of the cock were used as well. Women wanting sons were supposed to eat the testes.

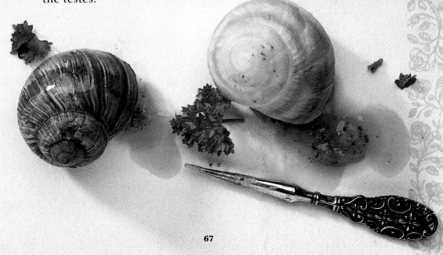

COCKLE BREAD

This charm has been used throughout Europe for thousands of years. John Aubrey (1627–97) described it as *"a Relique of naturall Magick, an unlawful Philtrum"*. The charm was made by young girls to attract a man, and consisted of a piece of dough which the girl had pressed against her vulva. The dough, thus moulded, was baked and presented to the man. If he ate it, he would be powerless to resist her. It was simple, inexpensive, home made and efficacious.

BIRD'S NEST

The bird's nest is one of the most powerful of Chinese aphrodisiacs, usually taken in the form of bird's nest soup. Rich in phosphorus, it is reputed to increase desire and improve erection. The birds which make these aphrodisiacal nests are sea swifts. With their gelatinous spit, they stick their nests made from seaweed to the walls of enormous caverns open to the sea. The caves where they nest are numerous throughout south-east Asia, in Malaya, Thailand and Java.

> *"Collecting the nests in semi-*
> *darkness with the stink from the*
> *droppings that cover the cavern floor*
> *is extremely dangerous work. It is*
> *like scraping a cathedral roof while*
> *balancing on a pole. There are two*
> *categories of nest. Black and white.*
> *The white nests are more expensive."*
> TOM STOBART, *The Cook's Encyclopaedia*

The nests are graded, the best being whole; the least good are simply fragments from the nest. They can be bought ready prepared, with instructions, from Chinese shops. The broken pieces are enterprisingly sold as Dragons' Teeth. Strongly spiced, bird's nest soup is reminiscent of French crayfish soup. This soup is expensive and the authentic kind is found only in high Chinese cuisine.

Bird's nest soup is also eaten in Europe, in particular in France *(nid d'oiseau)*, Germany *(Vogelnest)*, Italy *(nid di uccello)* and Spain *(nodo de pajaro)*.

LIQUAMEN OR GARUM

This was *the* aphrodisiac of ancient Rome, documented by Apicius. This manuscript is preserved in a 9th-century edition, now in the Academy of Medicine, New York. There have been reliable printed editions of his work in most European cities since the 15th century.

Liquamen, made from putrefied fish entrails, was considered an indispensable sauce when used in a moderate form, and a positive aphrodisiac in its strongest mixture. Pompeii was noted for its liquamen where it was made in the factory of Umbricus Agathopus.

It was also served with kid or lamb, sucking pig, hare and stuffed dormice, but invariably with almost all forms of fish and shellfish.

NUOCNAM

This potent Chinese aphrodisiac is remarkably similar to garum or liquamen and its origins are possibly as old. It is made from phosphorus, salt and decayed fish, spiced with garlic and pimento, and is available from Chinese food shops

---

Some Aphrodisiac Meals of Ancient Rome

Snails soaked alive in milk, mixed with wheat flour and roasted, basted diligently with liquamen, pepper and cumin.

Soft-boiled eggs pounded with pepper, lovage and soaked pine kernels with honey and liquamen.

Truffles boiled on skewers, then grilled lightly, and put in a dish of liquamen, after being pricked to absorb the liquid.

Mushrooms and tree fungi, served boiled, drained dry and covered with pepper and liquamen, lovage and honey.

Wild boar, cooked in the oven, with a sauce of pepper, lovage, oregano, pine kernels, myrtle berries, coriander, honey, wine and liquamen.

Venison, roasted lightly, and eaten with a sauce of pepper, lovage, caraway, celery seed, honey, vinegar and liquamen.

On the Seductive and Sensual Properties of

RAW FOOD

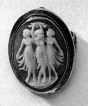

GOOD SEX NEEDS plenty of energy, and any depletion in mineral and vitamin levels in the blood undermines energy production and consequently the ability to perform the sex act. According to nutritionists, the average diet does not contain enough vitamins and minerals, and you need to find supplementary forms.

Raw food possesses far more vitamins than cooked food, from which the vitamins and minerals are leached in the cooking process. Vitamins that are water soluble, such as B, C, and E, can be lost in both preparation and cooking in water. Vitamins C and B2 are even destroyed by light. Peeling fruit and vegetables removes many of the nutrients that lie just below the skin, and proteins and fats are sensitive to heat. By eating fresh uncooked produce we not only obtain more nutrients but also avoid the additives contained in processed food.

For extra energy, and a better sex life, eat plenty of fresh fruit and vegetables, and drink ginseng tea.

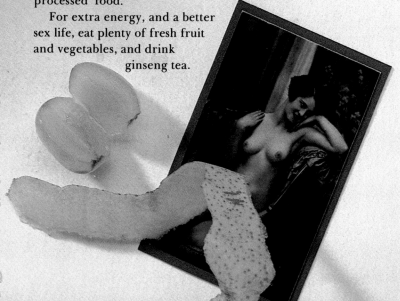

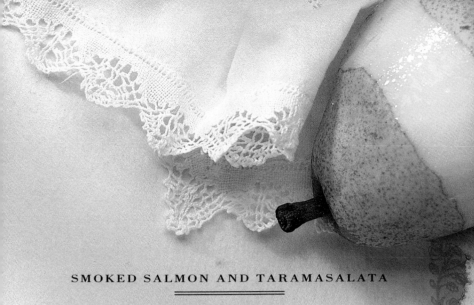

SMOKED SALMON AND TARAMASALATA

30 ml (2 tbsp) WHIPPED CREAM

50 g (2 oz) TARAMASALATA

4 SLICES OF SMOKED SALMON

8 cm (3 in) PIECE OF CUCUMBER

BLACK PEPPER, TO TASTE

1 LEMON

TO GARNISH: CRESS

Fold the cream into the taramasalata. Lay the slices of salmon on a board and spread with taramasalata.

Cut the cucumber lengthways into thin sticks and put a few on each slice of salmon. Season with pepper, roll up the salmon slices, and garnish with cress. Serve with a wedge of lemon, and brown bread and butter.

GREEK YOGURT, FIGS AND HONEY

4 RIPE FIGS

125 ml (4 fl oz) GOATS' MILK YOGURT

15 ml (1 tbsp) HONEY

TO GARNISH: FRESH MINT OR LEMON BALM

Slice the figs and cover the base of two bowls. Mix the yogurt with the honey and pour over the figs. Chill, add a sprig of mint or lemon balm, and serve.

71

JAPANESE FOOD

WITH ITS WIDE USE of raw fish and vegetables, Japanese food will do something special for you and your libido. *Unagi* (eel) considerably improves it, say the Japanese – there are 3,000 eel restaurants in Tokyo alone. The most special recipe is *kabayaki*, which is presented in a lacquer box (known as a *jubako*), with rice, soup and pickles all served separately. Eel is also served in many other ways – on bamboo skewers, with herbs, and in soup, for example.

The Japanese do not rely entirely on eel to turn them on. They also have *tsukemono*, which can add this facility to almost any food. Tsukemono is a pickle made in a remarkably similar way to the aphrodisiac of ancient Rome, liquamen. There are many *tsukemonos*, some more potent than others. *Shio uke* is made from radishes, gourds and cucumbers, which are put in a barrel and covered with salt. A lid with a heavy stone on it forces the juices out. Ginger pickle is *shoga zuke*; horse-radish and sake is *wasabi zuke*; the most expensive with the strongest sensual effect is *umeboshi zuke*, made, appropriately enough, from the plum, with its resemblance to the glans of a phallus.

Tempura is the Japanese way to eat fish by delicately deep frying it so that it is light and dry – making it very easy to digest. The *koromo* (batter) is made with iced water, and cunningly stirred to make it full of air bubbles. Japanese chefs never use the *koromo* twice and it is always as thin as paper, and transparent. When cooked, the *tempura* is dipped in a sauce or *tsukemono*, usually *daikon*, made with black sea-weed, white sesame seeds, almonds and cashews; purists, however, just dip it in sea salt.

FISH AND BAMBOO SHOOTS

1 CARROT, SLICED LENGTHWAYS, THINLY

2 THICK SLICES COD OR HADDOCK

250 ml (8 fl oz) DASHI OR FISH STOCK

15 ml (1 tbsp) SUGAR

45 ml (3 tbsp) SAKE OR MIRIN

30 ml (2 tbsp) SOY SAUCE (LIGHT)

125 g (5 oz) TIN BAMBOO SHOOTS

Boil the sliced carrot until just tender, put the fish and the stock in a wide pan and simmer for 5 minutes. Add the sugar, sake and half the soy sauce and cook until the fish is tender. Cook the bamboo shoots in the sauce for 3 minutes. In small bowls, place one piece of fish, some bamboo shoots and carrot slices, and add 1 tbsp of sauce.

UNAGI KABAYAKI (GRILLED EEL)

350 g (12 oz) FRESH EEL, SKINNED AND CHOPPED INTO SMALL PIECES

30 ml (2 tbsp) SUNFLOWER OIL

60 ml (4 tbsp) SOY SAUCE (LIGHT)

60 ml (4 tbsp) MIRIN OR SAKE

TO GARNISH: CUCUMBER OR RADISH

Flatten the eel pieces on a board using the blade of a large knife. Place the eel under a hot grill, brush with oil and cook for at least 5 minutes each side. Boil the soy sauce and mirin for a minute or two to make a glaze. Brush the eel with the glaze. Serve with finely sliced cucumber or radish.

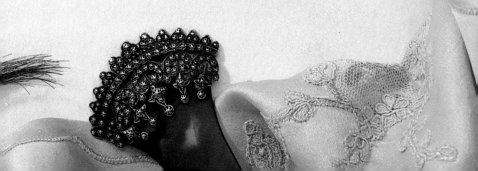

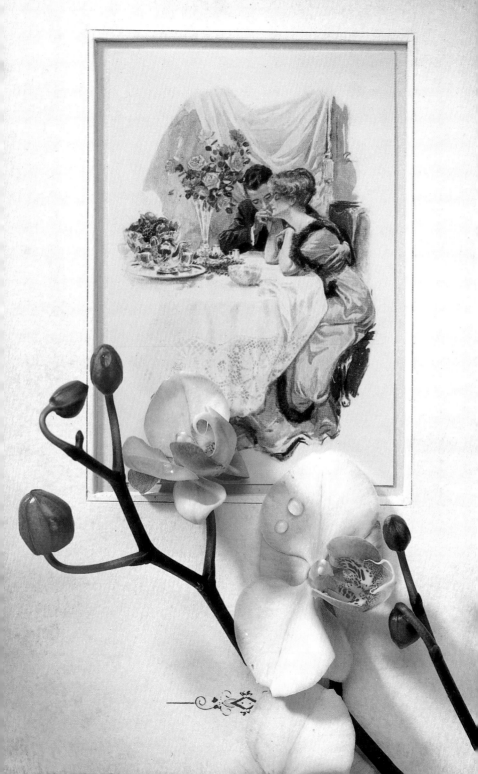

MENUS FOR ROMANTIC ENCOUNTERS

In Victorian and Edwardian times, in the
private booths of the great restaurants
where many an amorous encounter was illicitly
conducted, it was quite common for the couple to
be served as many as fourteen courses,
with a sorbet between each of the last three.
Fortunately, we are wiser than our grandfathers
and great-grandfathers. In this section I have
included some special menus for romantic
occasions and encounters which all heed the
advice that it is better to dine wisely, rather than
too well, if you wish the evening to end
with the same flourish that it began.
It is also important to make sure that the
performance of cooking the meal does not
impinge on your own later, and to this end dishes
have been chosen that are, by and large, simple,
quick and delicious, as well as being
great mood-enhancers.
A glass or two of wine will help to set the tone, but
beware of over-indulgence – it could well spoil
an otherwise perfect evening.

SPRING

"Welcome to Spring that moves men to love,
and you girls, inspiring your lovers,
yourselves made lovely with roses and
flowers, bred in spring hours."

ANGELO POLIZIANO (1454–94)

APHRODITE, THE GODDESS of love, had her chief festival on April 1st. To the Greeks (and the Romans, by whom she was known as Venus) Aphrodite was the generative force that pervaded the whole cosmos. Connected with flowers, sweet fragrances and female generosity, she rose originally from the foaming testicles of Uranus where they had been cast into the sea.

Springtime everywhere is marked by a procession of celebrations, from the old New Year on March 25th through to May 1st when the village maidens disappeared into the woods for a night and the May Queen married the Green Man.

If nothing else the folk lore reflects the human respect for creation and reproduction which is at the centre of the cult of Aphrodite, and naturally at its climax in spring. At this time of year the spirit and body are aroused to love and its consummation without stimulants of any kind, and lovers in spring time could reach the peaks simply on a drink of spring water and an apple.

MENU

PRAWNS IN GINGER SAUCE

ZARDA PALAU

ZABAGLIONE

～

The suggested menu for spring combines seafood, nuts, and eggs to
give you energy, but is suitably light for this time of year. The pilau
dish for the main course comes from Afghanistan and is very sensual
with just sufficient sustenance for an hour or so of exciting activity.
The zabaglione could be delayed until later as a restorative.

PRAWNS IN GINGER SAUCE

2 SPRING ONIONS, CHOPPED

SMALL PIECE OF ROOT GINGER, CHOPPED

15 ml (1 tbsp) SHERRY

15 ml (1 tbsp) GINSENG SYRUP

15 ml (1 tbsp) SOY SAUCE

4 LARGE PRAWNS, PEELED

SALT AND PEPPER

Place all the ingredients except the prawns in a saucepan. Bring to the boil and then simmer for 2 minutes. Put in the prawns, cover and cook for 3 minutes. Season to taste.

ZARDA PALAU

25 g (1 oz) BLANCHED ALMONDS

25 g (1 oz) PISTACHIO NUTS

30 ml (2 tbsp) OIL OR GHEE

1 SMALL ONION, FINELY CHOPPED

2 CHICKEN BREASTS, QUARTERED

5 ml (1 tsp) SAFFRON

125 ml (4 fl oz) LIGHT CHICKEN STOCK OR WATER

30 ml (2 tbsp) GRANULATED SUGAR

45 ml (3 tbsp) WATER

GRATED RIND OF 1 ORANGE

100 g (4 oz) LONG GRAIN RICE

Fry the almonds and pistachios in the oil or ghee and set them aside. Fry the onion lightly and set aside. Fry the chicken until golden, add the saffron and the stock and simmer for 20 minutes or until tender. While the chicken is cooking, cook the rice in plenty of boiling, salted water. When just tender, drain and keep warm.

Dissolve the sugar in the water, add the orange peel and boil to make a thick syrup.

Arrange the chicken pieces on top of the rice with the onion, and nuts, add the chicken liquid and finally pour the syrup over.

ZABAGLIONE

Use the recipe on page 23, with or without the satyrion, allowing two egg yolks per person, and adjusting the other ingredients accordingly.

SUMMER

S UMMER MEANS TRAVEL, freedom to escape day-to-day restrictions, adventurous forays into strange cuisine. The sun itself can be an aphrodisiac for some. Summer also offers the chance to eat out-of-doors; a moonlit meal on a balmy evening makes an ideal prelude to love-making.

MENU

GRAVAD LAX
LOBSTER AND MANGO
PEACHES IN RED WINE
—

This makes the most of summer bounty from the oceans and the orchards. Serve a good Chablis with the salmon, and a Puligny-Montrachet with the main course.

GRAVAD LAX

SALMON TAIL END, SCALED AND FILLETED	15 ml (1 tbsp) BLACK PEPPERCORNS, CRUSHED
15 ml (1 tbsp) SEA SALT	15 ml (1 tbsp) BRANDY
15 ml (1 tbsp) SUGAR	15 ml (1 tbsp) CHOPPED DILL

SAUCE:

30 ml (2 tbsp) GERMAN MUSTARD	100 ml (7 tbsp) OLIVE OIL
15 ml (1 tbsp) SUGAR	10 ml (2 tsp) DILL
1 EGG YOLK	SALT AND PEPPER

Make up the sauce as you would a mayonnaise, and set aside. Mix all the other ingredients except the salmon in a bowl. Rub the mixture into the salmon fillets, placing them one on top of the other on a board. Cover them with foil and another board and weight it down. Chill for 24 hours.

Drain the salmon carefully and slice it thin. Garnish with fresh dill and lime slices.

Serve with the sauce and slices of brown bread and butter.

LOBSTER AND MANGO

1 RIPE MANGO

450 g (1 lb) COOKED LOBSTER

8 SMALL COOKED CLAMS

FOR THE SALAD:

FRISÉE

RADICCHIO OR OAK LEAF LETTUCE

LAMB'S LETTUCE

60 ml (4 tbsp) FRENCH DRESSING,
MADE WITH WALNUT OIL AND
RASPBERRY VINEGAR

Peel and dice the mango. Dismantle the lobster, removing all the meat, in the usual way. Crack the clams, but leave them whole.

Arrange each plate with four clams and alternate slices of mango and lobster on a bed of salad, previously dressed.

PEACHES IN RED WINE

2 RIPE PEACHES

25 g (1 oz) SUGAR

2 ml (½ tsp) CINNAMON

300 ml (½ pt) RED WINE

TO SERVE: 125 ml (4 fl oz) DOUBLE CREAM

Peel the peaches, halve and stone them. Put them in a small pan with the sugar, cinnamon and wine. Bring to the boil, and simmer for 10 minutes. Take out the peaches, put two halves into each dish, and reduce the liquid to a syrup. Pour over the peaches, chill and serve with double cream.

Alternatively, serve fresh figs with some goat's cheese or Greek yogurt.

AUTUMN

S TALLS APPEAR on the sidewalk outside every other restau-
rant in Paris in September, piled competitively high with
oysters and any other shellfish you can remember. At this
time of year we seem closest to primitive man and to his
great oyster feasts on the beach, to ward off winter, and
ensure that as many babies as possible got off to a good start
the following spring.

Dizzy with shellfish and wine, and drawn to bed early by
the darker evenings, lovers can find autumn a particularly
sensuous time of year.

MENU

GINSENG SOUP WITH CHRYSANTHEMUMS
STEAK AND OYSTERS
PEARS BELLE HÉLÈNE

*For those intent on something more carefully organized, this menu
includes some sure-fire recipes for successful love-making.*

GINSENG SOUP WITH CHRYSANTHEMUMS

3 CHINESE DRIED MUSHROOMS	300 ml (½ pt) GINSENG SOUP
1 CHRYSANTHEMUM FLOWER	7 ml (½ tbsp) CORNFLOUR
100 g (4 oz) COOKED CHICKEN BREAST	1 EGG WHITE
300 ml (½ pt) BROTH	

Remove the stalks from the mushrooms and soak them.
Pull the petals off the chrysanthemum. Cut the chicken
into strips.

In a large saucepan, heat the broth, then add the ginseng soup and mushrooms. Simmer for 3 minutes. Add
the chicken and simmer for a further 3 minutes. Blend the
cornflour with a little cold water, stir into the soup and
simmer briefly, stirring. Whisk in the beaten egg white.
Pour into bowls and add the chrysanthemum petals.

STEAK AND OYSTERS

225 g (8 OZ) FILLET STEAK

8 OYSTERS

22 ml (1½ tbsp) SOY SAUCE

22 ml (1½ tbsp) OYSTER SAUCE

15 ml (1 tbsp) SHERRY

22 ml (1½ tbsp) VEGETABLE OIL

2 CLOVES GARLIC, CRUSHED

2 SLICES ROOT GINGER

3 SPRING ONIONS, CHOPPED

15 ml (1 tbsp) CORNFLOUR, BLENDED WITH A LITTLE CHICKEN STOCK

TO GARNISH: WATERCRESS

Cut the steak into two 1.5 cm (¾ in) slices. Remove the oysters from their shells.

Mix the soy sauce, oyster sauce and sherry. Add this sauce to the beef and leave to marinate for half-an-hour.

Fry the garlic, ginger and spring onions in the oil. Tip the beef and oysters into the frying pan and pour in the blended cornflour. Stir-fry for 1 minute. Serve on a heated dish and garnish with watercress.

PEARS BELLE HÉLÈNE

2 RIPE EATING PEARS

150 ml (¼ pt) WATER

15 ml (1 tbsp) SUGAR

VANILLA POD OR ESSENCE

150 ml (¼ pt) VANILLA ICE CREAM

SAUCE:

50 g (2 OZ) BITTER CHOCOLATE

25 g (1 OZ) UNSALTED BUTTER

TO GARNISH: 25 g (1 OZ) TOASTED FLAKED ALMONDS

Peel and core the pears and leave them whole.

Put the water in a pan large enough to hold the pears upright. Add the sugar and vanilla, bring to the boil and simmer for 5 minutes. Add the pears and poach gently until tender; leave to cool. Arrange on a serving dish and pour syrup over. Place a scoop of ice cream in each individual bowl, with a pear in the centre.

Melt the chocolate in a bain-marie. Add the butter to the chocolate in small pieces, stirring till the sauce is glossy, and pour over the pears while still warm. Sprinkle with toasted almond flakes.

WINTER

*"The winter wind
is like ginger."*

CHANG CH'AO

I N OUR GRANDMOTHERS' day, the choice of aphrodisiacs in winter was limited, the best sources coming from the spices and pickles that they used to preserve the summer harvest through the winter months. Nowadays, aeroplanes can deliver every ingredient we might need from all around the world.

Nevertheless, although we now have central heating, wall-to-wall carpeting, and instantly available ingredients, nothing quite replaces the quiet evening delights of a pile of cushions in front of a roaring log fire – the ideal time and place to serve up a hot posset made of warmed milk, flavoured with spices like cinnamon and cloves, and sweetened with honey.

MENU

GUACAMOLE
LAMB AND APRICOTS
BANANAS FLAMBÉ

—

*Filling and warming, without being heavy, this menu makes an ideal
prelude to a romantic winter's evening.*

GUACAMOLE

1 LARGE RIPE AVOCADO	2 SPRIGS OF FRESH CORIANDER OR PARSLEY, FINELY CHOPPED
15 ml (1 tbsp) LEMON JUICE	
1 TOMATO, PEELED AND CHOPPED	SALT AND PEPPER
¼ ONION, FINELY CHOPPED	1 ml (¼ tsp) GROUND NUTMEG
1 GREEN CHILLI, CHOPPED	

Halve the avocado and remove the stone. Scoop out the flesh, mash it with a fork, add the rest of the ingredients and mix. Cover the mixture with cling film and refrigerate. Use it the next day.

LAMB AND APRICOT

350 g (¾ lb) LEAN LAMB

25 g (1 OZ) BUTTER

2 CLOVES GARLIC, CRUSHED

2 ml (½ tsp) TURMERIC

2 ml (½ tsp) CORIANDER

2 ml (½ tsp) CUMIN

2 ml (½ tsp) GINGER

2 ml (½ tsp) BLACK PEPPER

2 ml (½ tsp) CAYENNE

1 ONION, SLICED

100 g (4 OZ) WHOLE DRIED APRICOTS, SOAKED OVERNIGHT IN 125 ml (4 fl oz) WATER

50 g (2 OZ) MIXED FRUIT OR SULTANAS

Cut the meat into cubes, melt the butter in a heavy saucepan and cook the meat until brown. Stir in the garlic and spices and add the onion and the apricot water.

Bring to the boil and then simmer very gently for 1½ hours until the meat is tender. Add the apricots and dried fruit, and simmer until the fruit is soft.

Serve with fresh dates, slices of fresh pear and rice.

BANANAS FLAMBÉ

2 ml (½ tsp) CREAM OF TARTAR DISSOLVED IN 300 ml (½ pt) WATER

2 LARGE FIRM BANANAS

75 g (3 OZ) BUTTER

60 ml (4 tbsp) BRANDY

SAUCE:

60 ml (4 tbsp) ORANGE JUICE

RIND OF ½ ORANGE, GRATED

60 ml (4 tbsp) WATER

30 ml (2 tbsp) BENEDICTINE

15 ml (1 tbsp) CURAÇAO

75 g (3 OZ) BROWN SUGAR

1 ml (¼ tsp) GROUND NUTMEG

Mix all the sauce ingredients and cook over a low heat until the sugar has melted. Put aside.

Mix the cream of tartar and the water. Peel the bananas and dip them in the solution. Cut the bananas across and lengthways into 4 pieces.

In a large frying pan melt the butter and fry the banana pieces, cut side down. Place the bananas in a chafing dish, keeping them hot, and pour the orange sauce over them. Warm the brandy and put it in a jug. Light the brandy at the table, pour it over the bananas and serve them while they are still flaming.

ANNIVERSARIES

"All kings, and all their favourites,
All glory of honours, beauties, wits,
The sun itself, which makes times, as they pass
Is elder by a year now than it was
When thou and I first one another saw:
All other things to their destruction draw,
Only our love hath no decay;
This no tomorrow hath, nor yesterday,
Running, it never runs from us away,
But truly keeps his first, last, everlasting day."

JOHN DONNE

The menu chosen here for anniversaries reflects the fact that they can happen at any time of year, and commemorate anything you want to remember.

The dishes included in this menu are fairly classical and will suit any occasion. Fortunately, these days, there are no limitations of geography or season as far as supplies of fresh produce are concerned. The recipes here are relatively simple and quick to prepare, so that, even if they are not prepared by the two of you, at least the one who is doing the work won't be much less fresh and enthusiastic afterwards than the other.

MENU

Globe Artichokes with French dressing
Filets de Sole au Champagne
Hot Spiced Apricots

—

Globe artichokes, which take very little preparation and have a proven record as an aphrodisiac, make a good starter for almost any choice of main course, followed by any of the fruits that are claimed to have special powers.

GLOBE ARTICHOKES

2 GLOBE ARTICHOKES

125 ml (4 fl oz) FRENCH DRESSING, WITH GARLIC

Cook the artichokes in plenty of salted, boiling water until the outer leaves pull off easily. Allow to cool. Cut the woody stem flush with the base. Serve with plenty of dressing.

FILETS DE SOLE AU CHAMPAGNE

2 FILLETS OF SOLE	¼ BOTTLE CHAMPAGNE (OR DRY WHITE WINE)
25 g (1 oz) BUTTER	
4 MUSHROOM CAPS	30 ml (2 tbsp) GOOD BRANDY
75 g (3 oz) MUSHROOMS, CHOPPED	45 ml (3 tbsp) DOUBLE CREAM
2 SHALLOTS, FINELY CHOPPED	2 EGG YOLKS
LEMON JUICE	CHOPPED PARSLEY

Season the fillets and roll them, skins inside. Melt the butter in a frying pan, add the mushrooms and shallots, and cook gently for 3–5 minutes. Set the four mushroom caps aside.

Add the rolled fillets, lemon juice and champagne, and simmer gently, with the pan covered, until the fish is cooked. Then transfer the fish to a serving dish and reduce the juices.

Combine the brandy, cream and egg yolks in a mixing bowl and add to the juices. Heat for a minute or two, but do not boil. Pour over the fillets. Add the parsley and the mushroom caps.

HOT SPICED APRICOTS

225 g (8 oz) APRICOTS, HALVED AND STONED	25 g (1 oz) BROWN SUGAR
	5 ml (1 tsp) CINNAMON
12 g (½ oz) BUTTER	60 ml (4 tbsp) ORANGE JUICE

Stew the apricots until tender. In a small frying pan, melt the butter, add the sugar, cinnamon and orange juice, and stir (with a wooden spoon) until the mixture forms a syrup.

Drain the apricots and add them to the pan, turning till glazed. Serve hot.

SAINT VALENTINE'S DAY

"Love's dwelling is in ladies' eyes
From whence do glance love's piercing darts,
That make such holes into our hearts;
And all the world herein accord,
Love is a great and mighty lord;
And when he list to mount so high,
With Venus he in heaven do lie."

GEORGE PEELE (*SONG FROM A MASQUE*, 1599)

Saint valentine's day as a love festival has no relation to the martyr of that name, but it is celebrated in many parts of the world by those in pursuit of love. Even the birds indulge in elaborate courtship rituals at this time of year.

MENU

Russian Egg Mousse
Duck with Chocolate Sauce
Tropical Fruit Salad

All lovers need the maximum strength they can derive.
The recipes here serve them handsomely. Wild duck tastes far superior
to the cultivated sort. Serve it with a simple green salad, and a good
bottle of Burgundy.

RUSSIAN EGG MOUSSE

3 EGGS	60 ml (4 tbsp) DOUBLE CREAM
5 ml (1 tsp) POWDERED GELATINE	2 ml (½ tsp) WORCESTERSHIRE SAUCE
300 ml (½ pt) CHICKEN AND VEAL STOCK	

TO GARNISH: A LITTLE CAVIAR

Hard boil and cool the eggs. Sieve the yolks, chop the whites and mix together.

Soak the gelatine in a little stock for 5 minutes. Mix with the remainder of the stock and gently bring to simmering point. Cool the stock and when the gelatine is thick enough, add the egg mixture and the cream and stir in the Worcestershire sauce.

DUCK WITH CHOCOLATE SAUCE

1 DUCK (MALLARD IF POSSIBLE)	⅓ BOTTLE DRY WHITE WINE
2 ONIONS, FINELY SLICED	BOUQUET GARNI
2 CARROTS, FINELY SLICED	50 g (2 OZ) DARK CHOCOLATE
15 ml (1 tsp) OLIVE OIL	JUICE OF 1 LEMON
60 ml (4 tbsp) WINE VINEGAR	BLACK PEPPER AND SALT, TO TASTE

FOR THE VEGETABLES:

100 g (4 OZ) EACH OF POTATOES, CELERY AND CARROTS, FINELY SLICED

30 ml (2 tbsp) BUTTER

Wipe the duck and prick it all over with a fork. In a flameproof casserole, gently brown the onions and carrots in the olive oil and set them aside. Place the duck in the casserole with the oil and brown it all over. Set it aside.

Put the vinegar into the casserole and heat until it is nearly all evaporated. Add the wine, onions, carrots, bouquet garni, seasoning and the duck. Cover and simmer for 1½ hours (or until the duck is cooked).

Take out the duck and joint it. Keep it hot. Skim off the fat from the casserole and stir in the chocolate and lemon juice. Put the sauce into a sauceboat and keep it hot.

Fry the mixed vegetables in butter in a large covered frying pan. Make a bed of them on a serving dish. Place the duck on top and serve with the sauce.

TROPICAL FRUIT SALAD

FRESH TROPICAL FRUIT AS AVAILABLE	60 ml (4 tbsp) LIQUID HONEY
30 ml (2 tbsp) LEMON JUICE	30 ml (2 tbsp) COINTREAU

Cut the fruit into small pieces, keeping the juices. Mix the remaining ingredients with the juices and pour them over the fruit.

On the Seductive and
Sensual Properties of
AL FRESCO FOOD

A WATERMELON AND a bunch of grapes fresh from the vine, shared on the roof of a ruined caravanserai in central Turkey; mellow blueberries staining our mouths in the mountains of the Haute Savoie; a large punnet of ripe Kentish strawberries on a shoulder of the Sussex Downs – picnics like these stay in our memories. On a hot day fruit is all you need for a lovers' picnic, but after a day in the driving rain on the hills of Skye, primus-stove-cooked porridge, washed down with malt whisky, makes an equally memorable and appropriate meal. The picnic itself is the aphrodisiac, and the primitive pleasure of eating with one's fingers is an appropriately sensual experience.

Seafood being one of the prime aphrodisiacs, no seaside picnic is complete without it. Clams are easy to collect, and among the best. There are recipes in Mrs Lincoln's *Boston Cook Book* (1891) for stuffed clams, pies and chowders.

Larousse covers every conceivable European way to deal with them, but the best way is over a camp-fire, right beside the disturbingly emotive sea.

Each country has its own special seafood. In France you might find the Venus shell, the Heart cockle or even the Warty Venus on your seashore. They can all be eaten raw, but they also make a delicious soup. In Ireland or Greece you might find sea urchins as a more exotic snack. Pull them off their rock, open them carefully, scrape out the bright orange ovaries, and eat them raw; they have the most sea-fruity taste there is. In Ireland they also cook them, treating them like boiled eggs: boil for four minutes, remove the prickles and the plug, scoop out the meat, and eat it with toast.

The snacks opposite are ideal for a quick burst of energy, when required.

CASANOVA SNACK

2 THIN SLICES ROQUEFORT CHEESE

4 SLICES PROSCIUTTO

4 THIN SLICES BROWN BREAD

Put a layer of Roquefort between two of prosciutto in each sandwich.

CHOCOLATE WALNUT SLICES

225 g (8 OZ) SHORTCRUST PASTRY	150 g (6 OZ) SOFT BROWN SUGAR
50 g (2 OZ) UNSALTED BUTTER	10 ml (2 tsp) STRONG BLACK COFFEE
100 g (4 OZ) WALNUTS	75 g (3 OZ) FLOUR
3 EGGS	

ICING:	CHOCOLATE ICING:
50 g (2 OZ) UNSALTED BUTTER	125 g (5 OZ) BITTER CHOCOLATE
150 g (6 OZ) ICING SUGAR	5 ml (1 tsp) CREAM
10 ml (2 tsp) STRONG BLACK COFFEE	12 g (½ OZ) BUTTER

Pre-heat the oven to 190°C (375°F), gas mark 5. Line a medium-sized shallow cake tin with the pastry and bake blind for 15 minutes.

Melt the butter, chop the walnuts, and whisk the eggs with the sugar and coffee until fluffy. Fold the eggs into the melted butter and add the flour. Blend in the walnuts and pour the mixture into the pastry case. Cook for 25–30 minutes. Leave to cool. Beat the butter, icing sugar and coffee until smooth. Spread on the cooled cake.

Melt the chocolate in a bain-marie and add the cream. Stir until smooth and add the butter chopped into small pieces. Stir until melted and smooth. Leave to cool slightly, spread on the cake and leave to set.

Cut the cake into squares. It will keep for several days in the refrigerator.

On the Seductive and Sensual Properties of

BREAKFASTS

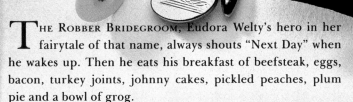

THE ROBBER BRIDEGROOM, Eudora Welty's hero in her fairytale of that name, always shouts "Next Day" when he wakes up. Then he eats his breakfast of beefsteak, eggs, bacon, turkey joints, johnny cakes, pickled peaches, plum pie and a bowl of grog.

In comparison with Marcel Proust's Madeleine cakes dunked in a bowl of milky white coffee in *À la Recherche du Temps Perdu*, this seems rather crude. Multitudes these days get by on orange juice and coffee, but this is no good for lovers who wake up dreaming of oysters and coddled eggs before rolling back to bed.

Wedding breakfasts should compare with Colette's. Hers included *"some small and melting hams cooked in a casserole, garnished with pink bacon and their own rind, bathed in their own stock, which was scented slightly with celery, slightly with horse-radish and slightly, too, with every healthy vegetable fit to be the aromatic servitor of such a mistress of that meat. We had crêpes too"*.

The following include a few suggestions that have a good supply of energy-giving protein.

HOT BUTTERED OYSTERS

Clean and open the oysters. Reserve the liquid. Toss the oysters in butter until hot through. Add the reserved liquid, plus extra butter to taste. Pour onto toast and serve at once with a thin wedge of lemon.

SCRAMBLED EGGS WITH SHRIMP

Scramble the eggs in the usual way, adding a handful of shrimps while the eggs are still runny. Season with salt, pepper and a scraping of nutmeg.

SALMON KEDGEREE

Mix together equal parts of cooked rice, smoked fish or poached salmon, and quail's eggs. Add a little chopped spring onion, curry powder and tomato sauce. Moisten with single cream, dot with butter and heat through thoroughly. Garnish with fresh parsley or coriander.

CODDLED EGGS

50 g (2 oz) SMOKED SALMON

4 EGGS

15 ml (1 tbsp) DOUBLE CREAM

TO GARNISH: FRESH CHERVIL, CRESS OR WATERCRESS

Butter two ramekin dishes and divide the fish, broken into small pieces, between them. Break two eggs into each dish and top up with cream. Put the dishes in an oven tin with water in it (to come half-way up the sides of the egg dishes). Cook in a moderate oven for 8 minutes or until set.

PRUNES IN WINE

These can be stored for up to a week in the refrigerator.

½ BOTTLE DESSERT WINE (BEAUMES DE VENISE)

1 LEMON, SLICED AND UNPEELED

100 g (4 oz) CASTER SUGAR

½ BOTTLE RED BORDEAUX

200 ml (⅓ pt) RASPBERRY JUICE

36 PRUNES

200 ml (⅓ pt) DOUBLE CREAM

1 ORANGE, SLICED AND UNPEELED

Mix the wines together and marinate the prunes in them overnight. In a large pan, the next day, add the remaining ingredients apart from the cream. Bring to the boil and simmer for 15 minutes. Store for 3 days in a cool place. Remove the citrus fruit, and serve with double cream.

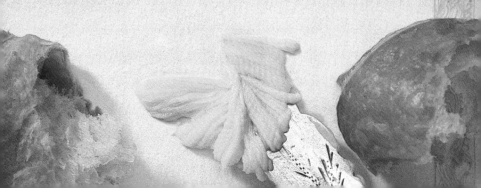

BIBLIOGRAPHY

APHRODISIACS

A. Comfort, *The Likelihood of Human Pheromones,*
Nature 239430, 1971
S. Fulder, *About Ginseng,* London, 1976
C. N. Hayter, *The Oyster,* USA, 1950
C. F. Leyel, *Elixirs of Life,* London, 1948
R. Lucas, *Ginseng,* USA, 1976
P. V. Taberner, *Aphrodisiacs, the Science and the Myth,*
London, 1985
Harry E. Wedeck, *A Dictionary of Aphrodisiacs,*
New York, 1989

SEX AND SEXUAL CUSTOMS

M. R. Anand, *Kama Kala,* Geneva, 1958
W. G. Archer, *The Loves of Krishna,* London, 1957
Sir Richard Burton (translator), *Ananga Ranga,* London, 1936
and *Kama Sutra of Vasyayana,* London, 1936
Jolan Chang, *The Tao of Love and Sex,* London, 1979
Seymour Fisher, *The Female Orgasm,* London, 1973
Germaine Greer, *The Female Eunuch,* London, 1971
B. Malinowski, *The Sexual Life of Savages,* London, 1929
Masters and Johnson, *Human Sexual Response,* London, 1966
J. J. Meyer, *Sexual Life in India,* London, 1952
Shayk Nefzawi, *The Perfumed Garden* (translated by Sir
Richard Burton and F. F. Arbuthnot), London, 1936
R. H. van Gulik, *Sexual Life in Ancient China,* USA, 1974

HERBAL AND CULINARY

Culpeper, *The Complete Herbal,* London, 1828
Alexandre Dumas, *Grand Dictionnaire de Cuisine,* USA, 1958
R. J. Farrer, *The Garden of Asia,* London, 1909
J. Gerard, *Gerard's Herbal,* London, 1957
T. Horoschak, *Walnuts,* Washington, 1972
D. E. Kester, *Almonds,* New York, 1929

C. F. Leyel, *The Magic of Herbs,* London, 1931, and
The Modern Book of Secrets, London, 1955
M. MacNicol, *Flower Cookery,* New York, 1967
N. T. Mirov, *Genus Pinus,* New York, 1967
P. Montage, *Larousse Gastronomique,* France, 1938
F. Rosengarten, *Edible Nuts,* New York, 1984
A. Simon, *Dictionary of Gastronomy,* London, 1962
T. Stobart, *The Cook's Encyclopedia,* London, 1958
C. E. Tuttle, *Chinese Herbs,* USA, 1956

GENERAL AND HISTORICAL

David Attenborough, *Life on Earth,* London, 1981
Simone de Beauvoir, *Old Age,* London, 1972
Colette, *Earthly Paradise,* London, 1952
Erasmus Darwin, *The Botanic Garden,* London, 1824
L. M. P. Foucher, *The Erotic Sculpture of India,* London, 1959
J. G. Frazer, *The Golden Bough,* London, 1890
Sigmund Freud, *Civilization and its Discontents,* London, 1933
G. C. Gillespie, *The Edge of Objectivity,* New York, 1960
V. Kaden, *Illustrations of Plants and Gardens,* V & A, 1982
P. & E. Kronhausen, *Erotic Art,* London, 1971
A. J. Smith (Ed), *John Donne,* London, 1971
Lin Yutang, *The Wisdom of China,* London, 1976

INDEX

ACKNOWLEDGEMENTS

AUTHOR'S ACKNOWLEDGEMENTS

Travel has been the basis for the manuscript and I am grateful to
my uncle, Captain William Urquhart, who knew and showed me
the China Seas and the Pacific. My constant companion in Europe
and Greece has been Joanna Stubbs, whom I must thank from the
heart. I must also thank Dr Joachim Fitzwilliam on Crete and Iris
Hennessy for all Irish recipes. For France, home of cuisine and so
many aphrodisiacs, Philippe Olivier, Dr Francis Scarfe and Dr Jean-
Pierre Benoist. For her help on medical matters I would like
to thank Dr Wendy Rostron. I should also like to acknowledge my
indebtedness to Jean-Pierre Shanjeux for his inspirational work
Neuronal Man The Biology of Mind.

PUBLISHERS' ACKNOWLEDGEMENTS

The publishers would like to thank Professor J.D. Phillipson of
the School of Pharmacy, London University, for checking the
manuscript, Barbara Croxford and Susan George for their
editorial help and Hilary Bird for compiling the index. Thanks
also to the following for their help with props for photography:
Elizabeth Corin, Wardrobe, Clive and Philip Antiques and the
House of Antiques, all of Brighton, Marston Barrett Ltd of Lewes
and Celia Allen of Battle.

The publishers would also like to thank the following publishers
for permission to quote: Martin Secker & Warburg and Farrar, Straus
& Giroux Inc. for the quotation from *Earthly Paradise* by Colette,
Batsford for the quotation from *The Cook's Encyclopaedia* by Tom
Stobart, William Heinemann Ltd for the quotation from *Venus in the
Kitchen* by Norman Douglas and Random House, Inc./Alfred A.
Knopf, Inc. for the quotation from *The Food of France* by
Waverley Root.